Optimizing Theories and Experiments

Randall R. Robey, Ph.D.
Communication Disorders Program
The University of Virginia
Charlottesville, Virginia

Martin C. Schultz, Ph.D.
Department of Communication Disorders and Sciences
Southern Illinois University–Carbondale
Carbondale, Illinois

Singular Publishing Group, Inc.
San Diego, California

Optimizing Theories and Experiments

Optimizing Theories and Experiments

Randall R. Robey, Ph.D.
Department of Speech Pathology and Audiology
Southern Illinois University–Edwardsville
Edwardsville, Illinois

Martin C. Schultz, Ph.D.
Department of Communication Disorders and Sciences
Southern Illinois University–Carbondale
Carbondale, Illinois

Singular Publishing Group, Inc.
San Diego, California

Singular Textbook Series
Series Editor: M. N. Hegde, Ph.D.

Child Phonology: A Book of Exercises for Students
by Ken M. Bleile, Ph.D.

Clinical Methods and Practicum in Speech-Language Pathology
by M. N. Hegde, Ph.D., and Deborah Davis, M.A.

Applied Phonetics: The Sounds of American English
by Harold T. Edwards, Ph.D.

Applied Phonetics Workbook: A Systematic Approach to Phonetic Transcription
by Harold T. Edwards, Ph.D., and Alvin L. Gregg, Ph.D.

Applied Phonetics Instructor's Manual
by Harold T. Edwards, Ph.D.

Communication Resources for Speech-Language Pathologists
by Kenneth G. Shipley, Ph.D., and Julie G. McAfee, M.A.

Also Available

A Singular Manual of Textbook Preparation
by M. N. Hegde, Ph.D.

Published by Singular Publishing Group, Inc.
4284 41st Street
San Diego, California 92105-1197

© **1993 by Singular Publishing Group, Inc.**

Typeset in 10/12 Garamond by So Cal Graphics
Printed in the United States of America by McNaughton & Gunn

Library of Congress Cataloging-in-Publication Data

Robey, Randall R.
  Optimizing theory and experiments / Randall R. Robey, Martin C.
Schultz.
     p.   cm.
  Includes bibliographical references and index.
  ISBN 1-56593-078-9
  1. Science—Experiments—Technique.   2. Physical measurements.
I. Schultz, Martin C., 1926–   .
Q182.3.R6   1992
507.2—dc20
                                                              92-25260
                                                              CIP

Contents

v

Preface

Hypothesis testing is the unifying centrality in all research employing experiments and quasi-experiments. Although one can examine or speculate about any interesting aspect of the world, one can have little assurance that the result of such mental effort will provide any sort of a reasonable map of reality. Further, assurance that the examination has led to a better or richer understanding comes through very few means. The most straightforward and scientifically acceptable understanding comes by formulating a cause-effect relationship and then making and testing a prediction of outcome from some set of antecedent circumstances. That is, one assures understanding by formulating a hypothesis and then putting it to test in an experiment or quasi-experiment. Whether through experiment or quasi-experiment, one increases his or her knowledge by structuring it carefully and testing it insightfully.

The rate of scientific advance is determined by an amalgam of (1) the quality of topical theories, (2) how insightfully experimenters focus the parts of the theory critical for advancing theory, and (3) how well the theories are realized as experiments, so that these parts of theory can be assured as the basis for understanding and predicting outcomes in novel situations.

This book deals with all constituents in the amalgam. It organizes theory by presenting a simple, coherent structure common to any; it charts the path from theory to hypothesis, putting one or more critical elements to test; it displays how to optimize each aspect of the design, implementation, and execution of an experiment so that the interesting hypothesis is put to test; and it maps the path from experimental result back to the model that is strengthened, revised, or rejected on the basis of the outcome of the test.

Section I provides the anatomy of theory allowing the researcher to move confidently to the critical prediction that becomes the research hypothesis. Section II delineates each stage of the realization of a critical research hypothesis within the limitations of an experiment or quasi-experiment, and Section III takes the reader back from specific outcome to theory with whatever change the result brings about. Although academic preparation in design of experiments and use of statistics is not prerequisite for comprehension, the book directly impacts the reader's insights into both.

This overall set of theory structures and corresponding realizations of experiments systematically centers on hypothesis testing as basic to all disciplines employing experimental approaches to acquire new knowledge. For this reason, examples have been chosen from a variety of disciplines, though familiarity (and comfort) has led to a preponderance of them in communication disorders and sciences and closely related areas.

In the interest of equity, gender references alternate across chapters; the researcher is female in even-numbered chapters. The order was determined by a flip of the ubiquitous unbiased coin. The ordering of authorship was likewise determined. Throughout the text, the letters in the first occurrence of each term appearing in the Glossary are capitals. There is some atypical grammatical phrasing; the specific occurrences and the rationale for adoption of each are discussed in text as they arise.

Section I structures the theory and experiment domains, and the correspondences between these domains become the bases for a discussion of experiment validities. The parallelism in structure is of primary importance for the interfacing of theories and experiments to optimize revision of theory, to the generalization of theory within a discipline, and to the integration of theories across disciplines.

Section II structures the experiment or quasi-experiment, including how to realize each constituent of theory. The section takes the experimenter from theory to and through the experiment, including everything from a choice of research hypothesis to development of conclusions from findings. Section II, in sum, organizes the considerations necessary for ensuring high quality in the experiment yield, as Section I lays the basis for ensuring high quality in establishing correspondences between nature and theory within experimental design.

Section II rationalizes the return to the domain of theory from the domain of the experiment for enhancing one's causal model or increasing its verisimility. The entire work cycles on itself, with Section III reopening consideration of the relationships among the domains and the implications for the scientific enterprise.

Acknowledgments

Earlier drafts of portions of the book have been read critically by colleagues and we thank all for their valuable contributions: Barbara Bain, Mary Ann Carpenter, Joseph Karmos, Kevin Kearn, Norman Lass, Dennis Leitner, Charles D. Parker, and Karl Perrin.

Most especially we wish to recognize Professors Alan Barton (Emeritus, Columbia University, Sociology), Sandra Ketrow (University of Rhode Island, Speech Communication), and Margaret Winters (Southern Illinois University, Foreign Languages and Literatures). Each provided specific and significant assistance to us on inadequacies in earlier portions of the manuscript. Ms. Terri Farris has been a wonderful resource throughout. The support and patience of Helen Robey and Beatrice Schultz passeth understanding.

We shall not cease from exploration
and the end of all our exploring
will be to arrive where we started
and know the place for the first time.

T. S. Eliot

1

Nature, Theory, and Experimentation

The Three Domains of Science

Science begins in observation of NATURE, the first domain. Although nature shows infinite variation, observers of nature believe that the variation is patterned. Scientific endeavor involves systematic study of the patterned (and nonpatterned) infinitely variable environment. To capture nature symbolically is to characterize through INDUCTION what is held by a particular culture to be the important or patterned essences of the reality.

Observations to capture the essences of the "blooming, buzzing confusion," contain more of interpretation than of description. Interpretation of observations presumes underlying regularities. These regularities produce what one observes and will produce something much like it again, one expects, following comparable antecedent conditions, events, states, or whatever. The basis for interpretation is the belief that universal regularities govern what we observe. Frequently, the goal of observation is creating the conditions to uncover such regularities.

1

Philosophy, in the last several decades, has seen a vigorous splintering including, of special concern herein, disagreement about whether the position we, the authors, espouse has either basis or utility. In the face of the philosophical difficulties, we defend a positivistic philosophy of empirical verification as being comfortable for many, perhaps most, physical scientists employing experiments for ensuring knowledge of the world. We believe that this same approach can lead to a deepening understanding of the behavioral and social sciences (BASS). In what appears to be an absence of alternative approaches to development of a unifying general explanation of the BASS, one either adopts a positivistic approach or abandons the development of general theory. But more than that, and in the face of the ambiguities, we believe that both the philosophical position and the pursuit of BASS development of generalized theory are sensible in that they yield, to a first approximation, useful results including a sense of deeper understanding.

Intellectual, or conceptual, modeling takes place in the second domain, the THEORY domain. From reflection on numerous observations, an explanation emerges. The combination of observations and explanation constitutes a theory, as we use the term. An alternative definition of the term, theory, is as an ideal or most rigorous form of scientific model. Theory thus defined constitutes some combination of laws, postulates, and axioms. Although we have no argument with those adopting such a philosophical position and rigorous definition, the "local" cost is the loss of the word for more general application. Therefore, we have chosen to define theory as the combination of observations to be explained plus some causal model.

Theories are organized to become progressively more useful maps of the regularities in nature. Further, because nature is believed to be the actualization of universal regularities, as theories evolve, they become progressively more universal. That is, theories fall into a natural hierarchy of progressively greater reach or broader inclusion.

The conceptual or theory domain, for POSITIVISTIC SCIENCE, is based in a set of assumptions: first, that the regularities of nature are robust, making universal explanation possible; second, the form for expressing those regularities in theory is Aristotelian-like. This means that nature's processes, whatever they may be, can be adequately mapped by statements formed from a deductive-like process. Third, theory cannot capture all of nature in manifest detail and it need not. All necessary particulars of nature must be captured in whatever classes or categories are deemed essential to any theory, but only the essences. Each class or category is conceptualized through arbitrarily determined dimensions for the salient facets of each essence.

At one time, fortuitous observation of events in nature that were critical as examples of positions or points was the only means scientists used to evalutate the tenability of theories, if done at all. In modern science, it is considered appropriate to put one's theories to test through observations of events by developing contrived microcosms of nature. For some time, scientists have manipulated nature directly through the medium of the EXPERIMENT, and the experiment is the third domain after nature and theory.

A word about some grammatical usage is in order. Appropriately, one should speak of "the domain of the experiment" or "the experimental domain." The first is the longer phrase but places focus on the experiment. The second is shorter and scans better in repeated appearances but places the reader's focus on the domain rather than on the experiment. For ease of scanning but appropriate focus, we have adopted the phrase "experiment domain" in much the same way political scientists discuss a nation-state.

In the experiment domain, one must realize all the important aspects of theory as expressing the essences of nature. Experimental constituents corresponding to all crucial aspects of theory are manipulated in a created microcosm of nature. As a result, the experiment and nature domains are distinct only conceptually. What distinguishes the two is that the constituency of the nature domain is found by happenstance, while the corresponding constituency in the experiment domain is systematically introduced by the researcher.

A theory includes postulated causal models for occurrences in nature. The causal models are formulated, rejected, and refined on the basis of more-or-less controlled observations of more-or-less controlled events in nature. Systematic manipulation of microcosms of nature to secure controlled observations are termed experiments. That is to say, the theory domain comprises best and ever-changing explanations of nature emerging from manipulated microcosms of nature.

The experiment domain comprises true experiments and quasi-experiments. All principles discussed in this book equally apply as well to quasi-experiments as to true experiments. The central commonality of experiments and quasi-experiments is the focus on hypothesis testing. The differences between the two relate to what portions of reality can and cannot be brought under control within a (quasi-)experiment. For ease of presentation, this work mostly discusses experiments, though the majority of applications may be to quasi-experiments.

Interrelationships Among the Domains

The *quality of experimentation* is a function of the integrity of the map of theory, that is, the correspondences of experiment to theory, with the *quality of theory* a function of the integrity of the correspondences of theory to nature. The dual linkages highlight the central importance of the correspondences among the domains and, as shall be discussed, there are few gatekeepers ensuring quality of correspondences.

The value of any experiment derives jointly from the quality of the correspondences of theory to the macrocosm and from the quality of the correspondences of the microcosms to theory. The first quality of correspondences determines the POTENCY of theory or indexes the utility of theory for furthering our understanding of nature. To illustrate: The statement, "Psychotherapy properly concentrates on having the patient clearly formulate his own goals, along with the actions he can take to achieve them," has greater potency than the statement, "Psychotherapy properly concentrates on having the patient understand himself."

Given that there is no objective means for establishing the explanatory power of a theory, potency connotes the utility of a formulation for advancing understanding. Potency, as we define the term for technical use, always concerns theory and its correspondences to nature. Further, the quality of an experiment is indexed by its potency: By how much is my understanding enhanced or clarified because of the experiment? This question is at the heart of all experimentation.

The second quality of correspondences, that of the microcosm to theory, determines the LEGITIMACY of experiments or the validity with which any topical theory is realized as an experiment. Moreover, once a researcher has settled on the most potent experiment he can conceive, he concerns himself with every facet of legitimacy to assure that the experiment as realized, conducted, and interpreted retains the potency originally introduced.

Potency presumes legitimacy, but legitimacy does not assure potency. That is, illegitimate experiments are not potent for advancing understanding, but legitimacy alone does not assure that an experiment will prove potent.

To learn about nature through experimentation is to follow a laborious route. A few specifics of nature are labeled as essential and generalized as characteristic and then expressed as their correspondences within the ideal domain of theory. Each theory is to capture these imputed essences of nature, including the underlying governing system controlling the appearances of the specifics. Each experiment is to capture the salient aspects of theory in eliciting a critical observation. Said differently, a theory is a best-possible distillation of perceived reality expressed in ideal terms, and an experiment is a best-attainable approximation of theory expressed in reality. Metaphorically, each theory purports to be a map of nature. The theory is transformed into a set of constituents realized within an experiment, thereby providing a direct inquiry into a microcosm of nature to determine the quality of one's understanding. As a theory is a map of nature, an experiment is a map of theory, or a map of a map.

The researcher's objective is to learn about nature, and the structured experiment is an important medium for learning. As indicated previously, assessing the quality of any experiment is not straightforward, because the linkages between the experiment and nature domains are mediated by theory.

Any proposed theory can only be evaluated through specific examples, i.e., manipulations in nature that are asserted to be critically representative of the conceptual ideal expressed by the theory. However, although the individual experiment is a part of nature, it is only more or less representative of the theory. The experiment captures the same causal mechanism purported to account for the original instance if, but only if, all the linkages from specific initial *instance* in nature to the *generalization* in theory to the specific experimental *instance* are of some arbitrarily chosen high quality. Moreover, as is discussed in the final chapter, every experiment is subject to the intrusion of chance in the realization of the particular experimental example to test the generalized and ideal theory.

Conclusion

In learning about nature from an experiment, a researcher develops a critical test and seeks universality of explanation, or cause, in nature for a valid generalization of particulars under specified circumstances. So the impossibility of assuring valid correspondences is tied to the impossibility of assuring valid inductive generalizations. In brief and perhaps arguably, therein are the challenges.

Section I

Introduction

Chapters 2 through 7 constitute the initial and theoretical section of this book. Chapter 2 lays out the elements of theory, Chapter 3 those of experimentation, and Chapter 4 those of the validities that monitor the correspondences between theory and experiment. Chapters 5 and 6 comment on the technology employed by researchers to obtain information, that carries some stated risk levels as to truth value, through querying microcosms of nature. Chapter 7 comments on some difficulties in developing insightful theory and in designing critical experiments.

2

An Anatomy for Theory

Constructing theory in science is a progressive process. The drive in developing explanatory schemes is toward progressively more generalized explanation. The implicit and the explicit organization is that of progressively bringing more breadth into the range of understanding and of justifying the increasing generality of structure. In this way, linkages are created within disciplines and progressively across disciplines. A collateral development is one leading to recognition and understanding of the influences that cause exceptional instances to deviate from a central uniformity.

Schematically, the evolving understanding of commonalities and also of exceptions takes place at the same time. Theory becomes more encompassing through more generalized explanation. For example, a theory may include a broadened population or environment to which it applies. A theory may become more detailed to provide the explanatory sophistication that leads to incorporation of previous exceptions. Any theory evolves primarily to an increasingly broader application and secondarily to an increasingly more specific set of explanations as to why, when, and how exceptions are to be found.

The bases of science are, on the one hand, a simple and universal set of fundamental elements of any theory and on the other, a belief in and accompanying drive toward being able to explain all phenomena within the generally accepted and universal theory. This explanation illuminates the relationships among the fundamental elements of theory. The acceptance of such an underlying conceptual scheme by many scientists is most apparent in the physical sciences. Historically, an extreme example can be seen in the Laplacian view that if the critical data were known about all the atoms that make up our universe for any given moment in time, then the locations for all the atoms for all successive moments would be completely predictable. According to this theory, the entire universe is held to be deterministic and conceptually predictable. Scientists have only to work until enough is known. Comparable motivations may power present efforts in the physical sciences to develop a grand unifying theory covering all phenomena.

A partial contrast can be found in current work involving Chaos Theory in a variety of the physical science (PS) domains. The contrast is only partial because, although chaos theory is based in the concept that both chance and the spreading effects of small and random occurrences may have large and unpredictable consequences, the consequences are consistent with the basic notion that one can encompass chaos within a theory.

Introducing chaos to any TOPICAL THEORY places some limits on the absolute resolution of that theory: Newtonian—that is absolute, static—laws will not suffice to explain all observed phenomena. Nevertheless, theory still serves toward some overall unification of all science. Whether one is prepared to believe in the possibility of a fully deterministic Grand Unifying Theory (GUT) or, rather, some approximation of a GUT that necessarily incorporates lawful indeterminacy, there seems to be little doubt that the progressive maturation of topical theory in all disciplines manifests an ever-expanding reach.

The authors are prepared to cover both BASS and PS disciplines by way of an example from physics because we hold that their organizational schema encompass common categories. Each branch of science holds a belief in a simple and universal set of structural categories and seeks progressively to formulate them.

Exampling the Challenge of Building BASS Topical Theory

Suppose a group of 20 or so researchers all sharing a common research interest is gathered together. Further, suppose that all are charged with advancing the state of their science, are informed that their individual efforts will be underwritten, and they proceed. At the conclusion of this project the products of the collected endeavors could be reasonably expected to advance the state of their science. However, if the researchers control the precise framing of their own hypotheses and if all other things are left to vary freely, it could be reasonably expected also that the collective product would not represent an optimal revision of whatever was the accepted theory.

For example, some research hypotheses are likely to be cast with distinguishing differences that constrain direct comparison. Also, there would likely be some incongruences, if not outright contradictions, among the findings. Perhaps the results of some studies would have appropriately led to revisions of other studies, had the former been completed first. One could certainly expect that an additional study, if not a series, would be necessary if the various findings are to be reconciled into a unified and coherent revision of the current topical theory.

The premise of this example is that when researchers pursue their own interests and all else varies by chance, theory will be revised and understanding will be advanced but neither will occur with high effectiveness or efficiency. Effective and efficient revision of topical knowledge comes through a guiding superordinate organizing scheme. Such an overall organizing scheme for advancing knowledge establishes the status of theory and indicates how to revise that status. An adequate overall organizing scheme shows how to advance knowledge in each science and how to integrate disciplines for a deepening understanding of the world and of ourselves.

How a Theory Is Structured

If any reasonably sized body of scientific literature is taken at face value, the volume of pieces of information that must be kept in focus can be difficult to organize. The process of trying to integrate what happened on this or that test administered under this or that condition to this or that group using this or that piece of equipment—let alone the need to reconcile these pieces of information with other findings—is at best a formidable task. Although the collectivity of all such findings composes the constituency of reality as we know it, the pieces of the collection are too specific and too numerous to explain reality. Some organizing scheme or theory must be superimposed or extracted to structure a more or less adequate explanation for what is otherwise a myriad of isolated details.

Two different manifestations, or levels, of universality are found in theories, because theories have a universal form and any one of the elements of any theory contains a universal class. At the first level, each theory comprises four ELEMENTS, which are CONSTRUCTS, ENVIRONMENTS, PARAMETERS, and POPULATIONS, plus a fifth component—CAUSE—describing the relationships among the elements. The theory element of populations, for instance, forms a universal class of all members meeting the criteria for inclusion, for example, all adult females with high school education or its equivalent.

All theories in the BASS share an additional type of universality: Each of the elements is characteristically unobservable in referring to a generalized conceptualization of, or a class name for, something that is known to exist but that cannot be seen in its entirety. Each can be referenced through exemplars such as: females, standard deviation, crowding, purchasing behavior.

Causation, which is the fifth COMPONENT of a theory, has a dynamic character and, therefore, is neither referential nor elemental. However, as is each element, it is a component of theory. That is, we have partitioned the structure of theory as comprising the four elements plus a fifth component that extracts the essence of the governing system in nature and thereby captures the causal relationships among the components. Whereas the *elements* of theory are different aspects of some phenomenon, the fifth *component*, causation, explains the basis for change(s) in their relationships. Consider each in turn.

Components of a Theory

Populations

Every scientific theory has population(s) as one element. A population is usually a very large group of entities or prospective observation units sharing a common feature or set of features. Often in the BASS, these entities are people. However, the entities may be entire classrooms of students, an animal species, a type of cell, or any other prospective observation units that may be objects of experimental interest.

A population comprises all of the entities in existence that example the common feature(s). For some purposes, a population may also include former and future exemplars of the features, e.g., persons becoming aphasic next week. Precisely which units are and which are not members of the population is determined by the population definition. At all times, the population definition is under the control of the theoretician/researcher and usually formulated to reflect her specific interests.

As any population definition becomes increasingly specific, more potential members are excluded progressively, and the size of the population diminishes. Consider the following examples of possible population definitional criteria:

Female
Stutterer
Severe stutterer
English speaking
Monolingual
Born and raised in the United States
Left-handed
Positive history of familial left-handedness
Postpubescent
Less than 20 years of age
Positive history of reading disability

Obviously, incorporating successive criteria from this list into a definition progressively changes the defining condition of the population and reduces its constituency. A population comprises all entities satisfying the definition.

Whether a population definition is appropriately broad or narrow is determined by researchers' interests in the modeling. The utility of a population definition as a piece of theory corresponding to some aspect of nature is an issue of precision. A precise definition clarifies membership for both identification and inference; a vague definition does not.

Unless a population definition is exclusive in the extreme, observing the membership is impossible. An example of extreme exclusivity might be the few people who claim to have witnessed a UFO landing at a specific location on some specified date. Setting aside this special case, the totality of a population is inaccessible, for example, E. coli bacteria, children in second grade. Although it is clear that such a totality exists, the overwhelming number of units dispersed over who-knows-where and who-knows-when makes direct observation of the collectivity impossible. Despite the inaccessibility of the total membership, one can observe a set or sets of examples and infer to the total membership. Researchers almost always seek to generalize a conclusion as applicable to all population members.

Constructs

A second element of any scientific theory is one or a set of constructs. A construct in the BASS is some property or process *attributable to each member* of a population. The property or process may be inherent as in hearing loss, behavioral as in communicative style, descriptive as in reaction time, or of some other nature. That is, a construct can be thought of as *an attribute that is characteristic of the population membership* the researcher is interested in explaining—behaviors, abilities, and percepts. When the population membership, that is the unit of observation, is larger than a single biological entity, the construct is likely more complex. As an example, consider the construct of Gross National Product in developed versus developing countries.

Examples of varieties of constructs in the BASS include intelligence, metabolism, job satisfaction, species adaptability, warfare, and a Bear market. In each case, the word or phrase connotes a concept or notion, but defies precise and universally acceptable definition. Moreover, people's impression of one of these terms may be reasonably but not completely uniform. It is a referent that likely is conceptually amorphous and probably varies somewhat in its conceptualization from person to person.

The nature of a construct is exemplified through the public debate regarding obscenity. The jurist who says, "I can't tell you what it is but I know it when I see it," expresses the nebulous quality of that construct in particular and of the nature of constructs in general.

Definitions of constructs are elusive and while aspects of nature recognized as interesting to BASS scientists, constructs are difficult to explain. There appear to be three essential characteristics to any construct in the BASS:

1. All constructs appear to be dimensional, occurring in greater or lesser magnitude;
2. The definition of a construct is criterion-driven: That is, the researcher must define which dimensions are to be included and over what range for each; and,
3. Quantification of the construct may require scaling processes that yield measures failing to meet the criteria for arithmetic systems.

All three of these characteristics essential to defining and to understanding constructs are discussed in detail, because the essence of explanation centers on constructs.

Environments

Environment(s), the third element, describes the temporal, physical, and social/affective contexts in which population members exist. Examples of environments include: a third-world economy, a clinic or classroom, presence of an "authority" figure, soil Ph, talking on the phone, time-pressure-inducing circumstance, and adverse signal/noise ratio. If the units of observation are collections of entities, such as nations, the environment broadens to become social/political/cultural ecologies. A large variance is to be expected across the experiences of population members placed in any of these environments. An environment, then, is a conceptual abstraction, a complex state that is for some reason(s) interesting, the influence of which cannot be observed and that is to be included in the theory.

Parameters

Parameters constitute the final element of any theory. Parameters are the medium for quantification because they are measures taken by necessity on populations. They index magnitudes of various aspects of constructs or relations among them in one or more populations within one or more environments. Examples of parameters include, μ, σ^2, ρ, and π. These specific examples are: population mean, population variance, population correlation coefficient, and population proportion, respectively.

This fourth structural element of a scientific theory, like the other three, is essential for universal scientific explanation of nature. Moreover, just as in the cases of populations, constructs, and environments, parameters are conceptual notions that are manipulated in the development of explanatory models of nature.

Causation

The final necessity for every theory is cause. Either implicitly or explicitly, the quest for a deeper understanding of nature often is found in the question, "Why is it so?" Although populations, constructs, parameters, and environments are necessary for describing some interesting aspect of nature, the fifth component of theory, which is the integrating relationship, is needed to provide the explanation for the interesting phenomena. CAUSATION, technically considered, offers an explanation for relationships among the elements and for changes in their relationships. More simply, causation is the researcher's conjectured explanation of whatever is sufficiently interesting that she asks, "Why is it so?"

Causation is the most elusive of the theory components because the explanatory scheme resides in the researcher. That is, the statement of cause has its genesis within the researcher's belief system. For example: "Every morning when I go to my desk to write, all my pencils are dull or have broken points, because, I believe, the Ploglies come out of the wall every night and recreate this existential state."

Explanatory schemes evolve in the early stages of exploratory research. Of course, absence of information and observations may preclude or limit any statement of cause. Early in an enterprise, a researcher's primary interest may be to determine the characteristics of one or more of the first four elemental theory components. If so, the researcher's belief system leading to some expression of causation depends on what is learned in the phases of the exploratory research.

As the researcher's sophistication grows concerning the aspect of nature under study, so does her sophistication about tenable causation. The initial product may be nothing more than a hunch. With repeated experimentation, the researcher gains sufficient insight to revise and refine some explanatory model for the accumulating observations. Eventually, the causal model becomes more formalized within some theory as the fifth component. Most frequently in NORMAL SCIENCE, the researcher conducts evaluation to promote a singular causal model. There are times, however, when one's need is to select among theories competing for primacy.

Competing theories often differ only in their expressions of causation. For example, consider two explanations for the genesis of neologistic paraphasia in persons with aphasia wherein the speech of the individual with brain injury contains frequent neologisms. Kertesz and Benson (1970) contend that the occurrence of neologistic paraphasia, an unrecognizable word, is the response of a disordered speech production mechanism, that is—some loss of the role of normally occurring inhibition of output language behaviors associated with loss of subserving neurons in instances of anomia. Anomia is an inability to retrieve a desired word. We term this an anomia theory. In contrast, Buckingham and Kertesz (1976) explained the occurrence of a neologistic paraphasia, an unrecognizable word, as a severe literal paraphasia, a distorted but recognizable word. By literal paraphasia, they mean the manifestation of neural code for a correct lexical selection which becomes perturbed. We call this a conduction theory.

Both theories agree on the population as persons with severe fluent aphasia, the construct as neologistic paraphasia, the parameter as frequency of occurrence, and the environment as conversational context. The theories are in opposition solely on the basis of causation. Agreement in the characterization of phenomena but sharp disagreement in explanations of the observations is a common occurrence in both the BASS and the PS.

Whether one of the two above statements of causation or some alternative is true, we cannot know. If a decisive or ideal experiment could be created, it might include technology capable of detecting and deciphering huge numbers of simultaneous cell functions, neural codes, and synaptic transmissions. But, even were the experiment to be accomplished, causation would still be inferred. Nevertheless, accumulating observations and advances in technology provide the basis for increased precision in causal models.

For the general case, cause can be conjectured but it can never be known. Still, pursuing the question, "Why is it so?" motivates much of our scientific endeavor. Although scientists may gather compelling evidence together, supporting even an elaborated statement of causation, such as: The light comes on when someone flips the switch because there is a power company generating electricity transmitted over wires that come into this building and are connected to provide necessary and appropriate energy to the light bulb, and including the presence of the flipped switch in one of the wires . . . , scientists cannot bridge the difference between the implications of evidence and any governing system in nature. Although technology may ultimately allow viewing the very essence(s) of life and of the universe, science can never prove what principles govern either.

Theory Statements

At best, models of nature arise on the basis of inductions. Although the generalization arises from specific episodes, the objective is for universality in the explanatory scheme. Therefore, it is not sufficient to describe the episode, but rather to extract and express its essences. The four elements of theory, constructs, environments, parameters, and populations, provide a structural base for that universality. The extraction of each essence arises out of dimensions arbitrarily chosen to capture the salient aspects.

Beyond expressing essences for any episode, the modeler must show how the four elements combine. Assuring the synthesis that offers universality of explanation requires unfailing systematic consideration of all elements. In model building, this need is met through a CANONICAL, or rule-governed, approach to synthesizing elements. We label the product of this *canonical* approach a THEORY STATEMENT. A theory statement is complete for purposes of creating a scientific theory. A theory statement is canonical in containing all four elements: constructs, environments, parameters, and populations; it does not however invoke an explanation, or cause. All theory statements must be formed to meet two conditions: The theory statement must be an active, declarative assertion and its negation must be open to empirical testing.

To recast the four basic elements common to any *why*, populations capture the *who*, constructs capture the *what*, environments capture the *where* and the *when* and under what conditions, and parameters capture the *how much* in the theory domain. All of these elements come together in a canonical, i.e., complete, theory statement.

A statement that does not explicitly detail every element may contribute to understanding but is not complete. The conclusion that more males than females stutter, might be the only salvageable conclusion from a particular study. However, the conclusion in making no mention of environments or parameters, does not satisfy the canonical criterion for a theory statement. The statement could be made a theory statement by explicitly mentioning such elements that are unknown; for instance, more males than females stutter by some unknown amount in undifferentiated environments. In this statement, the populations are female and male stutterers, the construct is stuttered speech, the environment is not specified nor is the parameter. At a later point in topical theory, the theory statement might evolve to: The severity of stuttering for adult male stutterers exceeds that for adult female stutterers by $\delta = 0.4$ (effect size) in all social conversations with strangers.

As is made apparent by the examples, a defining characteristic of a theory statement is that any statement becomes a theory statement only when empirical evidence allows the conclusion that its negation is untenable. As a concept, a theory statement presumes an ideal. That is, should a study result be suspect because of some threat to its validities, all competent researchers or theoreticians would appreciate the threat and reach identical canonical theory statements from the study.

We do not propose that observation is or can be theory-free. Rather, we suggest that evidence from any study result will be acceptable, if at all, only by those who accept a set of correspondences between nature and theory that provides meaning for the evidence. Therefore, those who accept the underlying correspondences of nature to theory and of theory to experiment should agree about the content of theory statements; those who reject the correspondences are likely to find the theory statements unworthy of any attention at all. The result of a general agreement about which inferences are or are not legitimately derived from the literature is that the set of theory statements composing a review and analysis of the literature should be the same from one reviewer to another.

The research papers that bear on any particular topic will be the basis for some set of theory statements. Each specific research paper may yield one or a set of theory statements that contribute to understanding of some research focus. For example, a factorial study of the stuttering of men and women in two environments may yield a theory statement about each main effect or the interaction(s).

Personal Theory

The term we employ for the explicit conceptualization incorporating the theory statements, plus the imposed value judgments of a researcher, plus the causal model of the researcher is PERSONAL THEORY. The collection of theory statements that relate to an individual's particular research interest composes part of the personal theory for that researcher. In addition, any personal theory also contains an explanation of relationships, or proposed cause, that the researcher chooses. Labeling it a personal theory is a recognition that the conceptualization may or may not have general acceptance; it is the individual researcher's structuring of the evidence—the theory statements—plus proposed explanation.

Various researchers will likely consider some studies more powerful or well directed than others by virtue of focus or potency or both. Each researcher assigns some merit rating to each theory statement based on its importance for her proposed explanation and incorporates the theory statement with its associated value into her personal theory. The definition of a personal theory subsumes the earlier definition of theory and adds the weighting the researcher assigns to the theory statements. The personal theory is the model on which experimentation is predicated. The object of experimentation is to promote, revise, extend, negate, and elaborate the personal theory. Topical theory, most often, is the personal theory of some researcher that has been accepted by others and, for the time, constitutes the more generally "received wisdom" about that segment of the discipline.

A personal theory not only pertains to a general research topic, but is concentrated on and organizes a specific research focus. Probably, the personal theories for two similar research foci mostly share common features. Whatever differences exist reflect differences in the research interests or in causal models or both.

A researcher's personal theory, then, reflects the status of the interrelationships of what is currently accepted concerning populations, constructs, environments, and parameters as each and all relate to a specific research interest. The interrelationships serve as the basis to explain what has been observed and perhaps to predict what might be observed or to control what will be observed. The criteria for a personal theory are that (1) it must account for all valid and germane observations, (2) it contain a causal model, however (im)precise, and (3) it must provide the basis for meaningful and testable hypotheses.

There will be times when two or more explanatory models purport to account for a given set of observations. In these cases, each causal model and the set of observations form a separate personal theory.

The researcher's organization of the data plus her explanation form her personal theory. Should she publish her personal theory with sufficient supporting data and warrant, her personal theory will likely form a significant portion of the focused topical theory. But at the time of her formulation and its publication, that theory, no matter how compelling, is personal to her. Only following general acceptance does the theory cease to be a unique responsibility of the individual researcher. By labeling her theory development as personal, we do not mean to imply any reduction in rigor of a warrant, but we do intend to maintain the conservatism of science. Scientific conservatism operates on the requirement that the individual researcher assume the burden of convincing the scientific community of the merit of her research and of her theorizing for personal theory to achieve acceptance. A personal theory is personal until it achieves the status of topical theory. The term personal theory also covers the topical theory that one incorporates into one's own explanatory scheme for revision or extension.

Extending the Coverage of Personal Theory

A systematic approach to building theory hierarchically begins in personal theory. Here all of the available information relative to a research interest is reduced to a finite set of statements, each containing the elements of theory. The canonical information is integrated into a more or less coherent model for explaining what has been observed and for predicting what might be observed. With acceptance, a published personal theory becomes part of topical theory and, in turn, contributes to the advance of theory in the discipline.

Systematic theory building occurs through three processes. Collectively these processes center on taking an inventory of what is accepted and what tasks are indicated for theory advancement. The first process is part of establishing topical theory, as has been discussed. The second and third processes are, respectively, the short-term and the long-term aspects of advancing theory. The short term aspect of extending the coverage of theory we term *Revision of Theory*, the long-term aspects we term *Scaffolding of Theory*.

Revision of Theory

The revision of theory at any level, including personal theory, is accomplished in a variety of ways. For instance, theory may indicate gaps or deficiencies that require experimental attention. A researcher may feel need for the extension of theory into unexplored populations or environments or both. Other researchers may feel need for the confirmation or, alternatively, partial revision of some theory.

Occasionally, a researcher may find theory wholly unsatisfactory. She may then attempt to show that it should be rejected on the basis of decisive observations that are inconsistent with current theory.

Ideally, she would do this by formulating a prediction that should not occur under accepted theory but that she believes will nevertheless occur. Completing the research program and confirming her belief, she revises theory by initially rejecting the current causal model. That same researcher or another may then offer a new causal model that accounts for all present and prior observations. The reader likely is aware that the concept of an observation being decisive in the BASS is an ideal and that a satisfactory decision regarding tenability cannot be made on the basis of a single inference.

Systematic revision of theory within the context of normal science is pursued partially through evaluation of inadequacies of the theory statements forming the content of theory. The researcher catalogs the detail of the set of theory statements. Some statements contain theory elements that are global rather than particular; other statements lead to potential hypotheses that are prospective theory statements. Some theory statements may present detail conflicting with that of other theory statements. Yet other theory statements may present information that cannot be integrated into a coherent theory because some necessary additional information is lacking. The catalog of these several types of obstacles to building a single, encompassing explanatory model for occurrences within the focus of interest is examined in revision of theory. The needs for clarification are rank ordered by the interests, and perhaps the experimental resources, of the researcher. The individual researcher examining this catalog of obstacles to a single, coherent explanatory model will be considering two questions simultaneously: What hypotheses does the catalog of inadequacies generate? and Which of these hypotheses is/are the most important if my chosen causal model is correct?

Scaffolding of Theory

Revision of theory encompasses proximal interrelationships in the components of theory: constructs, environments, parameters, populations, and cause. Scaffolding of theory deals with progressively more distal relationships, but the relationships involve the same elements. That is, scaffolding of theory at present provides the ties among elements that leads to integration of more distal phenomena, with these linkages to undergo future refinement. As a result, differing topical interests and even different disciplines are incorporated into progressively more encompassing explanatory models. The successful incorporation of theories is termed unification of theory.

Many physical scientists hold that all the physical sciences and, perhaps ultimately, all science will be unified into a single, encompassing Grand Unifying Theory (GUT).

Economies of Building Theory Systematically

The unsettled aspects of theory are more likely to be highlighted in a systematic approach to building theory than otherwise. The canonical structure of theory sharpens definition of unknowns and enhances the precision with which interrelationships can be predicted. On close examination, it becomes apparent that the exact form of some questions presumes the answers to other questions. Moreover, some predictions can be more precisely formulated as the answers to some of the questions become known.

Predicted ties among elements of theory provide the researcher with a mechanism for organizing a larger research strategy. That is, the bases for the prudent expenditure of resources and for efficient and effective means for advancing theory through programmatic research will be found in questions and predictions arising out of theory. We term the process for determining an optimizing strategy for integrating topical theories as scaffolding of theory. Such scaffolding progressively converges toward a single unified theory.

This presents dichotomous implications for constructing theory in the BASS. First, the quality of individual studies must be assured. Were the elements appropriately represented for their immediate purposes? That is, are the operational realizations of the constructs, environments, parameters, and populations appropriate for testing theory? But over and above these concerns, and presuming that they were all adequately rendered, the second concern is that the conceptualization of theory must be sufficient to the task of placing that theory into the evolving explanation of ourselves and the reality we inhabit. The theory must be coherent in and of itself and it must also fit with what else is known.

Most often an individual experiment focuses on a specific conceptualization of a theory, including a personal theory, and the realization and subsequent evaluation of the experiment occur within the frame of the theory. Programmatic research, by contrast, is organized from the perspective of fitting a personal theory and the experiment that is its realization into the context of a larger and deeper, unfolding explanation. Here, the initial considerations in the formulation of the personal theory are based in the desire to have results from specific experimental microcosms expand understanding of the larger macrocosm. Only after a scientist has been thoughtful about these more general linkages may she narrow her focus to the realization of a personal theory and from that to an experiment.

3

The Correspondence of Theory to Experimentation

R esearch is the process for advancing theory at all levels. Said somewhat differently, the objectives for research range from the advancement of personal theory to the progressive revision and expansion of topical theory. Mostly, BASS research takes the form of experimentation. Researchers go about the business of answering the research questions and testing the predictions given by personal theory. This means that one tests predictions or hypotheses arrived at through deductive-like reasoning by way of observations of reality.

Historically, this cycling from theory to experimentation to theory has posed problems for the BASS researcher. One reason for the difficulties has been insufficient structure in building, studying, and testing theory, particularly when researchers have not appreciated the need to consider all four canonical elements. Consequently, the relation of experimentation to theory likely has been subject to variation among individual experimenters at the expense of effective theory building.

Being sensitive to all four canonical elements, by itself, frequently results in expanded theory. Historians of science present numerous examples in which the inclusion or the particularization of one or more elements of theory has led to revision of theory itself. Some examples include the particularization of population, as in the prevalence of stress reactions or of heart conditions in African-American versus Caucasian-American persons, leading to enhancement of theory of disease processes in medicine. Alternatively, the particularization of environment, as in institutional versus residential placement for persons with mental retardation, has led to enhancement of theory of cognitive functioning in psychology and education.

A related problem has been that of trying to express intangible conceptual theory elements in reality. The elements of theory: constructs, environments, parameters, and populations, all ideals, must be expressed as the tangible elements of experimentation: VARIABLES, CONDITIONS, STATISTICS, and SAMPLES. In this isomorphism, each theory ideal has its corresponding realization in the experiment.

Two problems BASS researchers have faced in choosing these correspondences have been first, that the realizations in an experiment are necessarily less than or reduced from their ideals, and, second, that the realizations most likely introduce some dimensions, or facets, to the representation that are not of the essences of the theory elements.

Unfortunately, compromises are unavoidable. Consider examples for three theory elements. (1) Being unable to examine the entire population, a BASS researcher examines a collection of members of the population. (2) As the pertinent constructs can be neither observed directly nor defined in universally acceptable and exhaustive terms, a BASS researcher employs tests and the like to reflect some aspects of whatever the construct is. As a case in point, a researcher may choose to measure IQ performance, which is an experimental variable, as a (partial) representation of the theoretical construct of intelligence. Yet, the researcher is stuck with the fact that this choice, unfortunately but necessarily, will interject a related but confounding construct, that is, reading ability plus some unknown magnitude of measurement error. (3) Because the environment element of personal theory is an abstraction, BASS researchers often expose their subjects to a set of conditions they hope approximates the critical environment but which, in turn, may be subject to deleterious effects. And the same applies to choice of parameters.

Obviously, how well a BASS researcher develops the realization of each theory element dictates the usefulness of the experiment outcome for revising theory. The quality of the research design is defined, in part, by how relatively well or poorly a researcher represents the elements of theory.

Moreover, the means a researcher employs to represent the elements in some personal theory as experiment elements is a direct measure of validity of that experiment. Experimental validity in this sense is assessed on the basis of the definitions of theory components and the relative isomorphism of their representations in an experiment. The aspect of a research design that explicitly reduces a theory element to its representation in an experiment is termed the OPERATIONAL DEFINITION.

Operational Definitions

An operational definition specifies the experiment element corresponding to a theory element. That is, the operational definition states the explicit operations performed in capturing the theory element, a conceptual ideal, in some realizable form in an experiment. For example, one may operationalize intelligence in a human being by obtaining his score on an IQ test, but operationalize intelligence in a rat by measuring the time taken to run a maze. In adhering to a policy of using and listing operational definitions governing what essences of nature are to be examined within an experiment and how the examination is to be conducted, the researcher assures reliability and an openness to public critique of both process and outcome.

An experimenter's understanding and communication of a theory element and his representation of it show for the record how each theory element is operationalized for the explicit and exclusive purposes of an experiment. Said differently, through an operational definition one captures something that cannot generally be seen and embodies it within a simulation to systematically manipulate it within an experiment. Within a quasi-experiment, an operational definition captures a theory element without affording the opportunity for manipulation. The set of operational definitions providing these realizations within an experiment creates the microcosmic model of the personal theory. How powerfully that research impacts that personal theory is directly tied to the fidelity with which the EXPERIMENTAL MICROCOSM mirrors the theory.

Any operational definition is arbitrary, with determination of its content the prerogative of the experimenter. Other researchers, of course, might disagree with the appropriateness of any or all of how a given researcher might choose to realize a population, a construct, an environment, or a parameter. For example, one researcher may choose to determine health status by medical examination, whereas another may choose to determine it by examiner interview. In the final analysis, the utility and value of any operational definition must reside in the fidelity with which the resulting selection process realizes the element of theory that the process was designed to capture.

The final draft of an operational definition is a product of the researcher's belief system, both in its idiosyncratic aspects as well as how it is influenced by the scientific zeitgeist, the availability and limitations of measurement instruments, and the availability of resources such as time, personnel, or money. This often leads to even further operational definition compromise, with the theory element realized even more imperfectly than otherwise might be accomplished, for example, health status determined by neither medical examination nor examiner interview but by self-report questionnaire. For such reasons and other reasons as well, the utility of any experimental microcosm simulating theory is often disputed among researchers. Although it seldom seems apparent in these disputes, the fundamental issue often is not results but the quality of the isomorphism with which theory element(s) are represented in an experiment.

An experimenter may select operational definitions used by others (e.g., tests, statistics) or develop them for himself. In any case, justifying the selection is the responsibility of the individual conducting the research.

How the elements of theory and experimentation are tied together through operational definitions is illustrated in Figure 3-1. On the left in Figure 3-1 are the ideal but unobservable elements of theory. On the right are the corresponding, compromised but observable, elements of experimentation. The medium for moving from an unobservable element of theory to a realized element of an experiment is the operational definition. Optimal operational definitions lead to maximum encapsulation of elements of the experiment to their corresponding elements of theory and at the same time to minimizing the injection of nuisance effects.

Traditionally, only the operational definitions of constructs, realized as variables, have been explicitly and purposefully stated in BASS research. Appropriately but less often, the requisite information for operational definitions giving samples and conditions is found scattered throughout BASS research reports. The generally accepted format for reporting research serves to continue this unfortunate state. For the most part, operational definitions of parameters (i.e., statistics) are either not directly stated in BASS research reports or referenced to a supporting source. The reader thereby is left without full background to evaluate the quality of the correspondences between theory and experiment.

The operations resulting in each of samples, variables, statistics, and conditions are unique in structure. Each of the four types of

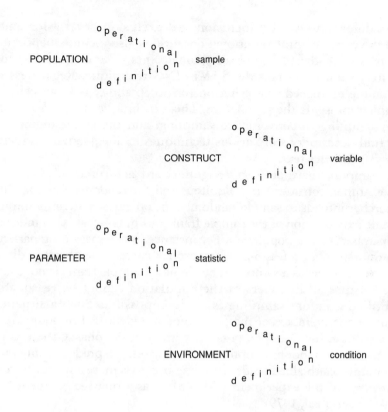

Figure 3–1 The roles of operational definitions in realizing elements of theory as experiment elements.

operational definitions requires a fundamentally different kind of information. They share a common purpose but, because each is unique, they are examined separately.

Samples

A sample is the representation of a population in an experiment. The population must first be defined to identify the desirable constituent members, exclusive of all nonmembers. To avoid potential confusions of population members and nonmembers, the experimenter must determine precise inclusion and exclusion criteria for entry into the experiment. Operational definitions also include mention of the means of identifying observational units. The method for unit identification is termed the SAMPLING technique. Regardless of technique employed, the criterion for acceptability is how well the sample represents the population. These techniques range from random sampling to convenience sampling, and the interested reader can find descriptions of various techniques in any good, introductory-level statistics text.

Sampling may not be so straightforward as is commonly believed. For example, consider the ubiquitous call for random sampling. If a researcher intends to sample randomly, the operational definition must include a description of the sample frame or limits—that is, an index of all members of the population. For instance, when measuring particular attitudes of a professional association, a current membership directory serves nicely as a sample frame. When a sample frame is not available because all members of the population cannot be reasonably identified, random sampling is made impossible. Such a situation occurs when members of the population are identified by some internal attribute, for example, persons with Broca's aphasia; there is no way to achieve random sampling. In such cases, the predominant situation in the health allied fields, sampling becomes more a matter of convenience and the experiment is described as a quasi-experiment (see Cook & Campbell, 1979).

Variables

Variables are the experimental representations of constructs. When a construct is to be manipulated, the variable is labeled independent. When a construct is observed for outcome, the variable is labeled dependent. Constructs to be mathematically controlled for their influence within the experiment are realized as variables termed covariates.

Regardless of the type of variable, achieving correspondence between variable and construct requires, first, definitions for both. Subsequent to defining both constructs and variables, the next issue to be decided is the scale of measurement. The well known scales of measurement, nominal through ratio, can be thought of as offering degrees of resolution in the *representation* of a construct, with nominal data being most gross and ratio data offering finest resolution. An extended discussion of scaling, including its requirements and its axioms, is in Chapter 10.

The degree of resolution that can be achieved is determined by a mix of an experimenter's interests and the limits of technology in representing the construct. An an example, consider cerebral dominance for manual performance, in other words, hand preference. Probably the least expensive measure of cerebral dominance for manual performance, to be registered on a nominal scale, is the answer to the question, "Are you right handed?" A better measure might be the response to the command, "Pick up that ball and throw it to me." However, since cerebral dominance is recognized as a matter of degree rather than type, an ordinal level index of the construct could be obtained using the Edinburgh Inventory (Oldfield, 1971).

A ratio level measure might be achieved, perhaps, if the multitude of all appropriate neurons could be observed directly and if the observations could be understood. In such an ideal case, absolute zero would be unequivocal nondominance that might be measured as equality of hemispheric neuron counts as well as function. Although the assumptions underlying the ratio scale example are likely never to be satisfied, better ordinal and, some people believe, better interval scale measures can be expected in the BASS as science advances.

Once the scale of measure is chosen for the operational definition of a variable, the researcher must determine if that single variable is sufficient to represent the construct. In some cases, a single representation is sufficient, for example, a 1960s representation of automobiles as being either domestic or foreign made. In other cases, a single measure is insufficient to capture the construct completely, for example, a 1990s representation of automobiles as being foreign or domestic, with the decision made on the dimensions of the assembly site, sources of ownership of capital, sources of component parts, and so forth. In this case, two or more variables are required, where each represents some unique aspect of the construct.

When a single variable satisfactorily represents the domain of a construct, the representation is univariate. A multivariate representation is one requiring two or more variables. Independent variables are usually unidimensional realizations of constructs. An exception occurs in the case of a statistical regression model where each predictor variable of a set may represent a different aspect of the same construct. Together, the predictor variables in such a set operationalize the construct. For example, SAT score, family income, and father's education might all be used to index academic potential as a way to predict GPA. Grade point average itself might serve as a variable indexing the academic achievement construct. An outcome construct may require one or more dependent variables to be satisfactorily represented. One or more covariates may also be required to achieve frugal representation of constructs.

Operational definitions also validate the selection of a variable as an appropriate embodiment of a construct on the bases of measurement validity and reliability. That is, the psychometric properties of a measurement device may demonstrably convince the reader that the device measures what it purports to measure, exclusive of unintended measurements—that it measures thoroughly what it purports to measure and that it is a stable index, for example, the *Wechsler Adult Intelligence Scale*, as perceived in 1960.

Statistics

Reducing parameters to statistics through operational definitions begins with defining the pertinent parameters and the pertinent relations among them. The definition of a parameter as pertinent in some ways dictates the unit of measure. For instance, if the parameter to be estimated is a mean rank, then the unit of measure must be a rank.

When the researcher operationalizes through a *descriptive* statistic, he must consider the mathematical properties of any estimator that pertain to its UNBIASEDNESS, CONSISTENCY, and relative EFFICIENCY. Discussion of these properties is in Chapter 11.

Application of an *inferential* algorithm is justified by meeting its mathematical assumptions. BASS researchers often have more than one algorithm available for assessing the tenability of a single NULL HYPOTHESIS. Obviously, the candidate algorithms may not be equally applicable to any given set of behavioral data. The researcher selecting the operationalization that yields an inferential statistic must provide a rationale for applying the algorithm. That is, he is responsible for making the case that the application will render valid evidence concerning an aspect of theory.

Conditions

The protocol for realizing environments as conditions must place inclusive and exclusive limits on the physical, temporal, and socioemotional aspects that are to be and are not to be represented. It must also address how complete and extensive the representations will be. The objective in operationally defining environments is to place observational units within specified conditions that maximally incorporate the environment of interest and maximally exclude the confounding, uninteresting, or unintended environments. The proper, or ideal, operational definition of environment assures fidelity between the observational unit's percepts in the experiment and the environment defined in theory.

The Reality of Designing Experiments

Although the reader must appreciate the need to achieve fidelity of correspondences, and equally so for all elements of theory, that is not the crux of our purpose. Rather, the germinal message is that an experiment must capture the essence of whatever portion of personal theory is to be examined through the canonical research hypothesis and its experimental realization. The experimenter must pare away all the nonessentials, all the nuances, for the experiment to illuminate, zero in on, and test the fundamental issues of a given personal theory.

Most often in the BASS, optimal operationalizations cannot be achieved. An experiment might simply be too small, resources too limited to achieve the totality of even that portion of theory under examination. What makes the circumstance even worse is that there are no rules for determining the elements of theory to be compromised first or those appropriate for most radical compromise. In one experiment or at some developmental stage of theory, for example, examination of the environments the theory is believed to cover may be most critical, as in the 1990 debate about the validity of cold fusion. If so, the environment(s) as represented within the experiment must receive first consideration and greatest protection against constraint or distortion. In the case of cold fusion experiments, first consideration must be given to avoiding contamination of the "experimental fluid" medium. In another experiment, perhaps no elements can be assigned priority. If so, each element of theory may be compromised in its realization, but one will do the best he can.

Finally, be prepared to discover that realizations achieved in experiments may differ from those originally intended by the experimenter. A full appreciation for the de facto compromises in the realizations of theory elements may occur only after the experiment is run. Overall, it should be obvious that the more compromised the experiment, the more narrowly drawn must be the resulting theory statements. For example, many experiments using college students as subjects may apply only to other college students.

4
Validity: The Correspondences of Experiment to Theory

In a formal sense and as an ideal, the relationship that experimentation must have to theory is that each element of an experiment include everything, but only everything that constitutes the corresponding element of theory. The quality of the correspondences linking the experiment and theory domains is referred to as the *validities of an experiment.* How potent an experiment may be for revising theory, then, is partially determined by the VALIDITY with which elements of theory are represented in the experiment. The validities of the correspondences are necessary for any experiment to be potent in influencing one's understanding. This means that there must be an explicit consideration of validity for each of the correspondences for the five components.

Several authors have carefully discussed validity issues in experimentation. These discussions define and provide examples of potential threats to validity as well as tactics to avoid problems. Among the most extensive and thoughtful is the presentation of Cook and Campbell (1979). The present discussion of threats to the validity of an experiment is largely derived from the Cook and Campbell work and offered in a much reduced form. Familiarity with the original is highly recommended. We seek to provide an understanding of the parallelism or isomorphism existing among categories of theory, of experiment, and of validity. Given that each theory component is expressed in a component of the experiment, the quality of each correspondence can be assured through a component of validity.

Cook and Campbell differentiated four types of validities: internal, statistical conclusion, construct, and external. The four validities qualify how well the experiment captures each of the five components of theory. The INTERNAL VALIDITY of an experiment speaks partly to the integrity of the face value of experimental findings. In addition, through internal validity one considers whether the independent variable(s) influenced the dependent variable(s) without concern at that time about the generality of either the influence(s) or the result. STATISTICAL CONCLUSION VALIDITY is to the integrity of the estimation of parameters. CONSTRUCT VALIDITY is the integrity with which the conceptual notions of constructs are represented as variables. EXTERNAL VALIDITY of an experiment refers to the integrity with which the two elements, populations and environments, are represented. The external validity of a prospective theory statement governs the populations and the environments covered by the statement. Because no study can satisfy all four validation classes in an ideal sense, the experimenter's task is to optimize across the four.

The parallelism among the categories of theory, experiment, and validity is displayed in Table 4-1. With the correspondences expressed by this schema in mind, we present some initial general comments, the coverage offered by Cook and Campbell, and their overall organizational logic.

In many ways, internal and statistical conclusion validities are in opposition to construct and external validities. Establishing causal linkages is most comfortably done within constrained circumstances—that is, with greater controls on statistical conclusion and internal validities. The narrower the design limits on sample, on context, and on the definitions of independent and dependent variables, the more likely one is to achieve success in establishing what Cook and Campbell term "covariation" (p. 37). The cost of constraining the experiment, however, is achievement of a very limited generalization on the observed covariation. By contrast, pursuing broad and universal generalizations by optimizing only external and construct validities likely increases error variance and reduces the chance of observing covariation. The experimenter confronts what appears to be a stand-off. Too great a concentration on statistical conclusion and internal validities more likely gives the desired effect but constrains the reach with which the researcher can generalize

Table 4–1 Correspondences Among Components of Theory and Experiment and the Associated Validities

Component of Theory	Component of Experiment	Type of Validity
construct	variable	construct
parameter	statistic	statistical conclusion
population	sample	external
environment	condition	external
cause	explanation	internal

her results. But, optimizing only external and construct validities may preclude obtaining anything but a trivial result.

While the difficulties in rank ordering the validities are not small, there is an implicit rationale to help make choices. Concern about validities is appropriate, because the validities ensure the legitimacy of an experiment. However, one invests in the validities of an experiment to assure legitimacy in support of potency. A lack of legitimacy undermines potency for theory revision; that is, a poor correspondence of experiment to theory can only result in a poor correspondence of theory to nature.

Value is maximized in achieving the most potent experiment a researcher can realize. The relative importances of the several validities are to be considered and ordered to protect the potency of the study. Recognizing the difficulties in reconciling the competing demands of these opposing validities, we present an expanded discussion of each.

Internal Validity

The internal validity of an experiment considers the accuracy of revision(s) of theory relating to causation. Two distinctly different circumstances need to be considered. One is the situation occurring in exploratory research where no formulation of causation yet exists. In this case, the claim of internal validity for an experiment is enhanced by ruling out nuisance agents that might otherwise generate misleading patterns in the data. That is, in exploratory research, although the researcher oftentimes need not know what caused the observed results, she must have some assurance about what did not cause them. The second situation occurs as the experimenter settles on some statement of causation, either formulated by her or adopted from elsewhere. In this case, the concern for internal validity centers on whether the observed outcome came about because of the posited causal relationship.

The metastatistical questions of causal relationship and of the direction of causality are the concerns of internal validity. The focus in examining internal validity is deciding if the treatment really caused the outcome. Threats to internal validity arise from occurrences within the experiment that can influence the outcomes or can call into question the coupling between treatment and measured outcome. Any events that may influence outcomes but that do not relate to the experimental treatment threaten internal validity. Tying treatment to outcome as stated in the research hypothesis is accomplished by ruling out alternative explanations for the results.

Consider examples of threats to internal validity. (1) Any influence or combination of influences upon subjects, for example, maturation of subjects during the time span of the study or repeated testing of subjects that leads to progressively sophisticated responses. (2) Influences on experimenters, such as progressive learning by the experimenter over the course of the study leading to a shift in criteria for categorizing responses. (3) An analogous change in any measuring device or instrumentation, such as change in calibration. (4) Difficulties of subject selection. Examples include extreme measures on subjects that may show ceiling or floor effects and likely will show statistical regression toward the mean in later testing or groups pre-experimentally may systematically differ on attributes that interact with the treatment variable. (5) Difficulties experienced in subject retention, such as when the experimental treatment causes a differential mortality in treatment groups, resulting in differing compositions of groups of subjects. (6) Studies with a different treatment to each of two or more groups run risks of having groups intercommunicate leading to diffusion or imitation of treatments, to some uncontrollable external equalization of treatments, or to a compensatory rivalry or a demoralizing rivalry between groups, or even to subject collusion aimed toward or away from the results desired by the experimenter.

In each case an invalid explanation placing responsibility for outcome on the treatment threatens the potency of any new theory statements and, subsequently, weakens the revision of theory in terms of causation.

Statistical Conclusion Validity

The legitimacy of an experiment for revising parameters within theory captures what Cook and Campbell call statistical conclusion validity. Legitimacy is the realm of the representativeness of one's numbers, the use of appropriate algorithms, and the correct interpretation of the product. Calculation serves to revise and extend the coverage of parameters in theory. The data collection process involves deriving numbers that will be used for estimating parameters and also for estimating relationships among them. The accuracy with which the estimates are formed from observations constrains the integrity of any revision of theory. Considerations of statistical conclusion validity form a significant portion of academic statistics curricula for BASS disciplines and are examined here only insofar as useful in an understanding of theory and its revision.

It is widely recognized that the validity of statistical conclusions is often at risk. The first threat to statistical conclusion validity that should be considered by the experimenter is the accuracy of the raw data. Then, she considers whether the assumptions necessary to the use of the chosen inferential algorithm are tenable. The stringency of this second requirement varies across tests but, as discussed in detail in Chapter 12, there are enough algorithms with differing assumptions to accommodate most data sets.

Following selection of an algorithm, additional threats to the statistical conclusion validity that are to be examined include TYPE I and TYPE II ERROR rates. Low reliability of measures may impact any experiment through the systematic misrepresentation of one or more elements of theory. Threats to statistical conclusion validity, as all threats to validity, are threats to the integrity of revision of theory.

A Type I error is a rejection of a true null hypothesis, whereas a Type II error is a failure to reject a null hypothesis that is false.

Group to group differences in experimenter conduct, in experimental setting, or other sources of heterogeneity may interact with some variable in the experiment. This may inflate the error variance or diminish the treatment effect. All these serve to decrease the legitimacy of revisions to theory. Not all of these occurrences fall exclusively within the province of statistical conclusion validity; for example, an increase in error variance because subjects differ in attributes that interact with the dependent variable(s) is an aspect of external validity. By way of summary, ensuring the integrity of the element of the experiment corresponding to parameters in the theory requires a careful examination of all threats to statistical conclusion validity.

Construct Validity

In the main, construct validity concerns the legitimacy of the relationships of variables in the experiment to the constructs of the theory. It is achieved through frugal, in other words, complete and economical, representation of constructs. The germane concerns are covered in statistics courses as *confounding* factors in experimental designs.

The major threats to construct validity are of underrepresentation, overrepresentation, and misrepresentation of constructs. Underrepresentation is caused by a lack of measures or operations leading to omission of significant dimensions of a construct. For example, examining learning disorders in children while measuring reading performance, the experimenter fails to measure mathematical, visual-perceptual, or auditory-perceptual skills. Overrepresentation occurs in the application of redundant measurement devices, as in the case of a researcher who estimates average hearing sensitivity by obtaining both tonal thresholds and speech reception thresholds. Misrepresentation, as implied, loads operations with irrelevancies, such as when one uses a test or questionnaire with unknown measurement validity and reliability.

Cook and Campbell's discussion covers the same issues in somewhat different terms. The tests proposed by Cook and Campbell for construct validity are: (1) that "independent variables alter what they are meant to alter"; (2) that "an independent variable does not vary with measures of related but different constructs"; (3) "the proposed dependent variables . . . tap into the factors they are meant to measure"; and (4) "the dependent variables . . . (are not) . . . dominated by irrelevant factors" (p. 61).

External Validity

Whereas the first three validities each deal with a single component of theory, external validity considers two: populations and environments. External validity is initially an issue of the legitimacy with which intended populations and environments are represented in the experiment. Additionally, whether findings can be applied to related populations and environments not represented in the experiment is a question of external validity.

While construct validity is typically introduced in statistics and design texts under the term "confounding," external validity most often is discussed as "limitations on statistical inference." Possible underrepresentation or misrepresentation challenge the legitimacy and therefore the potency of revision of theory for populations and environments. Can one generalize to the intended populations and environments with assurance?

Specific manifestations of threats to external validity are closely linked to manifestations of threats to internal validity. For example, interactions between treatment and differing subject groups with results that might systematically differ between different geographic, personality, gender, age, socio-economic, nonvolunteering, or otherwise characterized groups than those examined or sampled threaten generalization of the causal relation. That is, the willingness of the experimenter to generalize a valid causal statement to unwarranted populations or environments or both creates a common threat to internal and external validities. Can the result of a study on children raised with less restrictive parenting be generalized to children with more restrictive parents? Can the relationship be generalized beyond the laboratory or the school or the clinical facility? Can results from testing following a school-supplied lunch be generalized to performance any time during the school day by children from impoverished families?

Other threats to external validity include subjects performing atypically because of the special attention they receive as having been selected to serve in the experiment or because the treatment is seen as novel or special. Necessary initial or pre-experimental measures may influence later results by sensitizing subjects to the measuring device or instrument. In such a case, generalization to those not pretested is likely to be invalid.

There is a particular threat to validity that occurs across those disciplines addressing attitude creation, or attitude change, or behavior change. It arises from trying to balance resources and costs in an experiment such as conducting only short-term intervention when desiring to measure long-term change. For example, a treatment may create the conditions leading to emergence of behaviors or specific attitudes, but a need to complete the study before material resources are exhausted results in taking "final" measures before the final behavior, state, or manifestation could reasonably occur. Alternatively, for example, one may engage in a treatment that brings about some change at or exceeding criterion by experiment end. In both cases, what may be unseen and unmeasured is an extinction of the behavior or a change in attitude only occurring after completion of the experiment.

Final Comment

Historically, four types of validity have been identified. All facets of validity address the quality between the correspondences of the experiment and theory domains, elsewhere discussed as legitimacy. The elements of theory are not themselves independent and exclusive, as discussed in Chapter 7, so it should not be surprising that the validity classes also are not independent.

5

The Derivation of Potent and Legitimate Statistical Hypotheses

A change in personal theory is arrived at by modifying one or more theory statements, which may or may not alter the underlying explanatory scheme. That is, one enhances the data base or the explanatory scheme or both. This chapter discusses the underlying logic necessary for changing personal theory through experiments and quasi-experiments. Note that all statements necessary to altering personal theory reside exclusively in the theory or ideal domain—that is, they always involve generalization. The only constituents in each experiment domain are the realizations of elements within the microcosm of the experiment.

The anatomy for theory presented in Chapter 2 organizes the creation of theory from a literature review and segments it into two stages. The *first stage* is to capture a set of (canonical) theory statements incorporating the results from each study. Any theory statement makes mention of each of the four elements: constructs, environments, parameters, and populations. When an element is not explicated in a study, the researcher needs to mark it as unknown or undifferentiated. The collectivity of theory statements extracted through a literature assay thereby represents a

43

descriptive review. As such, the set of theory statements is to be one on which researchers working within a particular model agree.

The *second stage* occurs as the researcher introduces his insights, interests and creativity in synthesizing a set of theory statements into his particular personal theory. Which theory statements are more compelling, which are more suspect, which most important to the creation of his explanatory scheme? That is to say, while the set of theory statements is common across researchers, the personal theory that each person derives is likely to be unique.

Regardless of differences among personal theories, the primary purpose in establishing an individual perspective is to revise it. The contribution made by establishing a personal theory is that the researcher can then extrapolate beyond it. This section presents the structure connecting a personal theory to a tested hypothesis that will guide its revision. The structures throughout maintain canonical form to provide explicit consideration to all four elements.

Research Questions and Research Hypotheses

We define a RESEARCH HYPOTHESIS as a prospective theory statement with a RESEARCH QUESTION crafted to embody that assertion and its denial, which must be testable. First, examine research questions. Although What-if questions generated from implicit connections and expressed by analogy, metaphor, or other devices assist in the formulation of a research question, they do not qualify as such. Consider two examples of nonqualifying questions about personal theory. In the first, one might ask, "What would be the result if I used regime X and gave test Y to population P?" This does not qualify as a research question, because there is neither assertion nor denial. In a second, one might ask, "Is emotional counseling as effective as traditional psychotherapy?" Again, the question does not qualify as a research question, as the assertion rather than its denial contains an equality and therefore is untestable. For a question to qualify as a research question, it must embody a specific assertion, the negation of which is empirically testable.

Conservatism in science requires that a research hypothesis assert some change so that the null hypothesis is a test of its nonoccurrence. Within the logic of testing hypotheses, an assertion of equivalency is not testable.

If the initial interest is a speculation on the *reach* of theory, the route to changing a personal theory leads to a research hypothesis. While research hypotheses and research questions are both extrapolations of theory, the research question frames either of two alternative outcomes, with the research hypothesis predicting a single effect. A research hypothesis is a statement that if accepted *extends* one's present theory by adding a new theory statement to it, whereas a research question is more likely an inquiry about *inadequacies* in current theory. That is, a research hypothesis is a statement that accepts present theory and prospectively extends it, whereas a research question is more likely an inquiry that challenges present theory.

Research questions are important because the route to theory change beginning with questions is more likely to lead to unexpected knowledge than is the road beginning with hypotheses. Questions offer better opportunity than hypotheses for the play of intuition, creativity, and luck. Examining our own questions keeps motivation and inherent interest high. Certainly, re-examination of the *rationale* of a paradigm is more likely to follow from research questions rather than from research hypotheses.

Research questions and research hypotheses are instruments of theory. As such, they make no mention of things like groups, tests, significant differences, or any other aspects of experiments.

Research hypotheses are prospective theory statements, but become theory statements only through experimentation. As prospective theory statements, research hypotheses must be formulated in accordance with the rule-governed structure for theory. Further, because a research hypothesis is one outcome of a research question, the research question also must be uniformly expressed in canonical form. Although research question-driven revision of theory is more likely to lead to unexpected results, research-hypothesis driven experiments are more likely to be critical and therefore can best impact theory. Each form contributes uniquely toward changing personal theory.

Research questions evolve from initial interest in the *adequacy* of personal theory, while research hypotheses evolve from initial interest in the *reach* of personal theory. When sophistication of personal theory motivates the enterprise, a research hypothesis is likely to be the form of the expression leading to theory change. When the utility of personal theory itself is at issue, the perspective on changing theory likely leads to a research question.

Personal theories give rise to any number of research statements, some in the form of research hypotheses and others framed as associated research questions. Some are more likely apparent to the researcher and others less so. In some conceptual sense, as the researcher tries to determine which experiment he should run, he must contemplate all the individual research statements within a set of indefinite size. Settling on one or more good research statement(s) is more difficult in the early stages of paradigm development than in later stages. The development of theory through programmatic research is the progressive refinement of research statements, along with the introduction of altogether new perspectives as they become apparent.

Critical Research Questions and Critical Research Hypotheses

No matter how many research statements a researcher contemplates, the experiment he chooses to run should arise out of the research statement he sees as most critical for his personal theory. However, what research statement is most critical need not be determined on the basis of priority. Achieving optimum correspondences to the essences of nature as represented in theory elements, that is, potency, is a fundamental requirement for achieving critical experiments.

A critical research question or hypothesis focuses most directly on challenging the researcher's explanation of nature. Two kinds of criteria, then, may assist the search for the critical research statement. First, the research statement may be critical because it is fundamental to alternative research statements. This means that the answers to one or more fundamental questions may have to be determined before other research statements can be effectively formulated. Second, a research statement may be critical because it has maximal potency for revising theory.

The researcher entertaining *more than one personal theory* chooses his critical research hypothesis or critical research question from a broader set of candidates. Here the critical research statement must be selected from among the research statements of *all* considered personal theories. The likely choice will be the research question or research hypothesis that simultaneously and most substantially affects the plausibility of all the theories.

Statistical Hypotheses

The two statistical hypotheses, that is, the null hypothesis and the alternate hypothesis, by conventional wisdom, are mathematical expressions of quantifiable relationships among *variables* and are meant to apply to designated *populations*. The alternate hypothesis affirming the effect is prefaced by: H_A. The null hypothesis, that holds that the relationship expressed in the H_A does not exist is prefaced with the symbol: H_0. The conservatism of science requires that the pair of statements be written as mutually exclusive and exhaustive and that the tenability of the null hypothesis be evaluated. In the interests of optimizing BASS research to maximize its potency, statistical hypotheses are always written in canonical form by detailing all four elements.

When the usual form of the null hypothesis is examined, it can be found to contain an element of theory (i.e., parameters) and an element of an experiment or reality (i.e., variables). To say that differently, research hypotheses and research questions include only ideals, but null hypotheses and their alternate hypotheses each include ideals (i.e., parameters) as well as operationalized approximations to ideals (i.e., variables for constructs). This distinction is essential because null hypotheses cannot be tested on constructs, but theory cannot be built on variables. Researchers must necessarily test null hypotheses expressing variables, but their interest is in conclusions expressing constructs. Moreover, statistical inference requires that the experimenter concern himself with parameters and not statistics, so that null hypotheses mix theory and experiment elements.

One additional comment. The statistical hypothesis is generally of the form: H_A and not-H_0, so that its connection to explanation is covert. However, when the expression of the statistical hypothesis is prefaced by the causal component, the logic of hypothesis testing becomes transparent. That is:

IF (cause), THEN H_A and not-H_0;

or, alternatively,

BECAUSE (cause), H_A and not-H_0.

In texts, it is commonly recommended or taken for granted that hypothesis testing occur through direct translation of a research question to a null hypothesis. We believe that this implementation provides no sense of process and too frequently produces an ineffective product. Even at best in the use of this strategy, the scientist's attention regarding the foundation for revising theory is misdirected through focus on the absence rather than the presence of the experimental effect. A better understanding of the steps in the process comes through examining each stage of development from the research hypothesis to the null hypothesis that will actually be tested in the experiment .

The path from personal theory to the tested null hypothesis routes the experimenter from research hypotheses—or research questions to their research hypotheses—to the critical research hypothesis. Once dimensions of all elements in a critical research hypothesis are set, the researcher translates the statement to a mathematical expression termed the PRIME HYPOTHESIS (H_P). A transformation is then carried out on H_P to create a realizable, albeit less universal, expression termed the ALTERNATE HYPOTHESIS (H_A). The transformation is achieved by substituting variables into H_P capturing the dimensions of constructs and of environments. Each H_A is then evaluated in terms of both potency and legitimacy: the potency of the critical research hypothesis and the legitimacy with which the potency is preserved in the face of the necessary introduction of experiment domain elements. Note, however, that the experiment domain elements are expressed as ideals. Moving from the prime to the alternate hypothesis changes the basic form of the expression from *parameters of constructs for populations in environments* to *parameters of variables for populations in conditions*. Once formed, the expression of the alternate hypothesis is negated to yield the null hypothesis (H_0) to be put to test.

For reinforcement of the process of structural sequencing, consider a rewording. A mathematical translation of the critical research hypothesis takes place and results in an ideal mathematical expression, the prime hypothesis, comprising only theory elements including constructs. The alternate hypothesis (H_A) is a diminution of H_P, with the generally agreed on operationalized realization of constructs as variables, and also the less often discussed and often not operationalized realization of environment as conditions. The tested null hypothesis (H_0) is then formulated as the logical denial of H_A. All stages in the process, whether verbal or mathematical, need to be annotated for all four types of elements.

Ultimately, all theory elements of the critical research hypothesis must be realized as experiment elements. The dimensions of populations and parameters likely define the experimental realizations. For instance, if central tendency is dimensionalized as a mean, then the corresponding statistic is a mean. Further, a population of male left-handed registered voters should correspond directly to the analogous sample composition. In both cases, what is left for manipulation is the form of implementation: for example, WINDSORIZED MEANS and systematic sampling following a randomly chosen starting point.

Although the dimensions of populations and parameters lead to classifications that make the theory-to-experiment correspondences rather direct, the same is not true of constructs and environments. Those dimensions are likely interdependent continua, causing the theory-to-experiment correspondences to be rather indirect.

An Example of the Sequential Process

The generally accepted logical sequence of research hypotheses to null hypotheses serves to accentuate that the foundation for theory revision is the research hypothesis. Consider an illustration of the process. The sequencing is:

Research hypothesis: average academic achievement of undergraduate students in urban universities who are residing in nonuniversity housing exceeds that of undergraduate students who are living on campus.

In this research hypothesis, the construct is academic achievement, the populations are students living in or not living in university housing, the environment is undergraduate universities in urban locations, and the parameters are means.

The prime hypothesis takes the form:

$$H_P : \mu_{AA_{UUU_{\overline{UH}}}} > \mu_{AA_{UUU_{UH}}}$$

where $\overline{UH}$ denotes not-university housing. The verbalization of the prime hypothesis is: mean academic achievement of urban university undergraduates living off-campus exceeds mean academic achievement of urban university undergraduates living on-campus.

The construct: academic achievement, is indexed by the single variable: grade point average (GPA).

The alternate hypothesis is written:

$$H_A : \mu_{GPA_{CU_{\overline{UH}}}} > \mu_{GPA_{CU_{UH}}}$$

The alternate hypothesis is verbalized as: mean GPA of City University undergraduates living off-campus exceeds mean GPA of

City University undergraduates living on-campus. Achieving the H_A as a realized experiment requires a realization of every theory element. There must be clear definitions for urban universities and a sampling procedure for on-campus and off-campus living and a sampling procedure for populations of subjects under each living condition and a sampling procedure and so forth.

The null hypothesis is:

$$H_0 : \mu_{GPA_{CU_{\overline{UH}}}} \leq \mu_{GPA_{CU_{UH}}}$$

The null hypothesis is verbalized as: mean GPA of City University undergraduates living off-campus does not exceed mean GPA of City University undergraduates living on-campus.

Conclusion

The relationship of research hypothesis and alternate hypothesis is as direct as it can be, given the compromises necessary to make possible the experiment, which requires transforming theory elements to experiment realizations. The alternate hypothesis is the compromised form of the prime hypothesis, but it is the prime hypothesis and not the alternate hypothesis that is one of the two alternatives in the dichotomous research question inquiry. By contrast, the relationship of research question and null hypothesis is only indirect. The null hypothesis is the negation of H_A, but not the negation of H_P. Therefore the null hypothesis and the research question are not logically connected and neither can be deduced from the other.

An advantage of canonical and logical hypothesis testing is to maximize the correspondence between intentions and outcome from two separate perspectives. First, to be as specific as possible about one's expectations so that one can evaluate the match on outcome. The second is to focus on the elements of one's theory and one's experiment to assure that the correspondences are specific and legitimate. The first advantage addresses potency in applying the intended explanation to nature—that is, the relation of theory to nature. In this regard, the process moves through the formulation of research hypotheses as expectations based in the best current knowledge and culminates with direct evidence for the tenability of the expectations. As a result, specific expectations relate to specific null hypotheses, and nonfocused or general expectations translate to omnibus null hypotheses. The most pitiful cases arise when a researcher bypasses any logical examination altogether and empowers an equation, for example, an *F* ratio, to define the tested null hypothesis. In this worst case situation, it is possible for the researcher to test null hypotheses that are completely outside the point of the personal theory being examined.

The second linkage between intention and outcome focuses on the legitimacy of the intended correspondences of experiment to theory elements. This second linkage is particularly important in transforming prime hypotheses to alternate hypotheses where constructs are rewritten as variables. Because the constructs that interest BASS scientists are often external manifestations of complex internal events, constructs are most often best represented in multivariate form. The canonical application of the logic of testing hypotheses brings a recognition that constructs and variables are not isomorphic. The objective in the translation of H_P to H_A is complete but frugal representation of constructs as variables. That is, the objective is to obtain optimum representation of the construct with the smallest set of variables. When the problem is multivariate, maximum potency for theory revision can be obtained only through evaluation of multivariate null hypotheses. And, just as one must take care to ensure construct validity, so must he take care with the representation of the other theory elements.

NORMAL SCIENCE, which is practiced to assure high quality in empirical result, holds to a fundamental dictum that care in process is necessary, if not sufficient, for high quality. Logical hypothesis testing, which centers on the sequencing from theory elements to experiment outcome, provides clarity so care can be taken in the total process from literature review all the way to evaluation of the tested null hypothesis. With appropriate care, the canonical null hypothesis, even more than being an extrapolation out of personal theory, is a crucial step toward its revision. It may now be apparent that when the alternate hypothesis is framed, the *experiment* is largely structured; when the null hypothesis is framed, the *analysis* is likewise structured.

A frequent misrepresentation of the logic of testing hypotheses holds that the experimenter believes the null hypothesis to be true, that is, that testing of the H_0 is a position statement on theory unless evidence suggests otherwise. Of course, this is not the case; rather, scientists are impassioned human beings driven by belief systems. Initial focus on research hypotheses provides an avenue for expressing the implications of a scientist's beliefs without biasing outcomes. Canonical application of the logic of testing hypotheses loads *meaningfulness* onto the alternate hypothesis and, as a result, the evaluation of the complementary null hypothesis becomes a critical test of the researcher's theoretical position. It is notable that a single rejection of the null hypothesis on the basis of a probability no more validates the presence of an effect than a single failure to reject establishes its absence.

6
True Experiments and Quasi-Experiments

A researcher intending to change the state of theory by testing some hypothesis necessarily conducts some form of experiment. Modern science holds that *true* experiments require random selection and random assignment of observation units from a single population. Otherwise research hypotheses are put to test in quasi-experiments.

Although there are clear distinctions to be made between true experiments and quasi-experiments, throughout most of the book no distinction is drawn; both are considered within the class: experiments. In this chapter, the distinctions are important. All three categories: true experiments, quasi-experiments, and the general term, experiments, are dealt with specifically, and the discussion is couched in terms of values and costs.

Once the experimenter has defined a population, no matter how well or poorly done, the requirements for a true experiment constrain her decision prerogatives. She must meet requirements on sampling to represent the population and the mechanics of assigning observation units. The experiment must meet the condition that, initially each group is an independent microcosm of a common population and what differences exist prior to the experiment are properly attributed to chance. This is a necessary attribution for the use of algorithms developed on the assumptions of random selection and random assignment. That is, the mathematical proofs for these algorithms were written for the conditions of true experiments. The value secured through meeting these constraints is assurance of optimum correspondence between populations and samples. The primary value of a true experiment, then, is the inherent assurance on parameter estimation, which translates to assured validity of statistical conclusion.

By contrast, the risk levels for inference are unknown when the conditions of the proof are not met, even though the outcomes of robustness experiments have demonstrated the utility of some algorithms beyond the assumptions necessary to a true experiment. Unfortunately, the character of critical research hypotheses in the BASS likely precludes satisfying the stringent criteria for a true experiment. Because the quasi-experiment does not have the same assurance about parameter estimation as does the true experiment, the experimenter conducting a quasi-experiment has the responsibility for assuring *all* aspects of validity.

The researcher opting for a true experiment diminishes her burden of establishing the value of the experiment, even though none of the other validities is influenced by the more stringent requirements. For example, while the parameter estimation requirement establishes independent groups, maintaining that freedom from contamination of the direction and magnitude of the effect—threat to the internal validity—is a task required of the researcher. The researcher must also strive to achieve adequate correspondences in transforming constructs and environments as variables and conditions.

While the value of a true experiment resides in assuring some aspects of its legitimacy, its potency—the critical quality of the research hypothesis—is unaffected by its being a true experiment. That is, while potency presumes legitimacy, which is at least partially assured in the true experiment, potency is wholly determined by the composition of the critical research hypothesis. The overriding principle is that one optimizes experiment design to preserve the potency of the critical research hypothesis, independent of the form of the experiment itself.

The value of true experiments is the inherent assurances they give on some aspects of external and statistical conclusion validities.

A critical research hypothesis must be transformed to a structured microcosm of nature satisfying the criteria for true experiments in order to assure that value. But consider the implication of satisfying these criteria, given that critical research hypotheses in the BASS often preclude such precisely controlled microcosms. For example, researchers often have to compare populations distinguished by inherent attributes of the memberships, thereby precluding random assignment. In the frequently occurring case that a true experiment is not possible, the only way to satisfy the criteria would be to alter the critical research hypothesis to a less than critical form. That is, assurances on some aspects of external and statistical conclusion validities would come at the expense of potency.

The analogous cost in quasi-experiments is a sufficient investment of thought and resources to assure all theory-to-experiment correspondences are of high quality. But, in contrast to a forced true experiment, these expenditures yield a return. The value of quasi-experiments is an inherent potency of critical research hypotheses in the BASS.

Consider the issues within a larger context. The purpose of experimentation in normal science is revising personal theory through critical research hypotheses. The *highest value in design of any experiment*, then, is maintaining the critical research hypothesis. In the BASS, critical research hypotheses most likely demand quasi-experiments rather than true experiments, because it is unlikely in the BASS that one can employ random selection and random assignment and still retain the critical research hypothesis. So while achieving the highest value most often demands conducting a quasi-experiment, the quasi-experiment exacts the greatest design expense from assuring that all correspondences preserve the potency. By contrast, to go cheap and not assure legitimacy exacts a price in diminished potency; valued ends are not attained through cheap means.

The distinction between true experiments and quasi-experiments has so far been based on the former being open to manipulation for random selection and random assignment and the latter less or not at all open to such control. There are additional distinctions to be drawn. Examination discloses two stages in organizing any quasi-experiment. First, the researcher must seek an exemplar or exemplars for the experiment, for example, which type of ant colony under what circumstances will I choose? Having chosen, the experimenter can then introduce whatever manipulation, if any, she can bring into constructing the microcosm.

Control over construction of the microcosm diminishes progressively across the range of endeavors from the true experiment to the extreme of natural observation, such as occurs when anthropologists

immerse themselves in Caribbean cultures to enhance their understanding of coup stick rituals as aspects of societal behaviors. As one
moves from choice of a quasi-experiment, which is closer to a true
experiment, toward a choice closer to naturalistic observation, the
importance of induction increases in specifying the relationships of
theory and experiment elements. At the extreme of naturalistic observation, the induction produced by the observation is not unlike the initial induction following the observation that prompted the paradigm.

Conclusion

The design of any experiment germinates from the critical research
hypothesis. The potency of the research hypothesis rather than the
form of the experiment is the sine qua non. Often, in the BASS, the
critical research hypothesis requires a quasi-experiment. It is mostly
more difficult to assure legitimacy in the quasi-experiment than in
the experiment so the costs of legitimacy are likely higher. Potency
presumes legitimacy, so these costs must be borne in the interests of
the potency of the critical research hypothesis.

7
The Reality of the BASS

This initial set of chapters, together with their functional relationships, has laid out the idealized structures necessary to optimizing experimentation in the BASS. To restate: nature is mapped as theory and theory is realized as experiment. The tasks of the researcher are to create a theory corresponding to nature and then an experiment translating the theory. The microcosm that is the experiment serves as the medium for directed questions and responses that will progressively strengthen the ties from theory to nature.

We have proposed that theory be formulated through a five-component system: cause, constructs, environments, parameters, and populations, which captures the essence(s) of nature. However, in all of science there exist no external criteria for establishing the truth value of theory, as there are no external criteria for establishing the existence of any external reality (nature). Within the BASS, we obtain evidence of only the *perception* of external reality, with evidence for reality only indirect. Troubling or not, indirect evidence is the best one can get; shy of this, there is no evidence.

Research encompasses the loop from theory to experiment to theory. Whether one is thoughtful in going from theory to experiment or not, the reality of the experiment constrains the generalization from experiment to theory. This chapter elaborates on the complexities and challenges of BASS theorizing, examining the nature of theory elements, theory statements, and of personal theories.

Characterizing the Essences of Nature

Theory is a medium for communication. The creation of theory follows from one or more motivating observations of nature. An observation is captured in the theory domain by relating it to self and perhaps to others. An initial task in theory creation is expressing the morphology of such an event in ideal terms. We term the salient aspects of the observation as essences-of-nature and purport a fourfold classification of the terms of the ideal: constructs, environments, parameters, and populations. The completeness and precision with which an observation taken from the domain of nature is related to self determines the potency of the expression. Obviously, potency is compromised by incompleteness of expression or errors of omission, and imprecision of expression or errors of commission.

But how are completeness and precision of expression achieved? The answer begins in the process of characterizing perceived reality through chosen dimensions. Expressions of all four types of theory elements arise out of the dimensions underpinning each. For example, the parameter, "mean," is a location on the dimension of central tendency, whereas "variance" is a location on the dimension of dispersion. In general, the expression of each type of theory element: constructs, environments, parameters, and populations, arises out of some dimension that has been tacitly arrived at and then is explicated for the purpose of communicating perceived reality. Whether the final explicated dimension is formulated by self or adopted from others is a matter of prerogative. But, whether formulated or adopted, every explication unavoidably carries some set of dimensions for each theory element.

In the BASS, the interesting essences of nature likely are multifaceted. If so, the analogous theory element is multidimensional. For an expression to be potent requires that each principal or cardinal facet and no others be insightfully dimensionalized. The expression must be complete and precise. An experimenter must confront, first, whether he has discerned the explicit dimensions that he needs for each theory element and, second, whether he has achieved the fineness of resolution he needs on these dimensions.

The four theory elements become invested with distinct characters as dimensions in the experiment domain. The dimensions underpinning expressions of parameters and of populations lead to apparent classes of substructure. As a result, expressions of parameters and of populations are characterized as *definitional,* in the sense that they can only be exampled for purposes of constructing a microcosm of nature. By contrast, if the dimensions underpinning expressions of constructs and environments lead to classes at all, they are much less apparent and much more ambiguous. Expressions of constructs and of environments are characterized as *dimensional* because their counterparts in the experiment domain are likewise dimensional, albeit approximations.

As the discrepancy increases between the intended dimensions and the dimensions that actually arise out of the microcosm, the quality of the correspondences between the experiment domain and the theory domain deteriorates. That is, errors of omission or dimensions not realized at all and errors of commission, which are impoverished or confounded representations of intended dimensions, as well as representations of extraneous dimensions, all compromise validity.

Researchers in the BASS are often quick to adopt an existing measurement device in designing an experiment. Such a decision can be wholly satisfactory. However, when one adopts an existing variable, one accepts the dimension(s) that it captures. That is, operationalizing always determines the dimensions of one's elements. Given that dimensionalizing will occur, don't do it thoughtlessly.

The Character of Theory Elements

A difficulty in constructing theory in the BASS is that one must try to capture some *state* that is indefinable for being internal to the subject, such as intelligence, or otherwise intangible, such as culture. We call the intangible a construct and appreciate that the construct is an ideal, not totally capturable in words and likely even less well realized as a variable through measurement device(s).

Environments are yet more ephemeral than constructs. Although environments are external states, their transforms are indexed not on the external state but on one's perceptions of those external states. The perception is an admixture of the external state and the reactions of the observation units to the state. This admixture provides the experiment element conditions that corresponds to the theory element of environments.

Experimenters can struggle to control the creation of external states designed to motivate specific perceptions or classes of perceptions, but they have no direct assurance on control of the observation unit's perception of reality. That is, exercising scientific control over experiment conditions can be very difficult because the experimenter cannot control the perceptions. Further, the only insight possible about the effect comes from measuring the observation unit's response to a directed inquiry by means of some quantified index. The influence of the environment is captured *only* as it alters the observation unit's response(s) to the perception. The theory element of environment has not generally been considered carefully in research design literature and, likely, environment is the element given least attention by researchers.

There are no conditions-free observations. The theory element of environment is always realized as experimental conditions, even when the experimenter considers it to have no influence on the internal state or construct. The influence of environment in experiments is always expressed in the measurement that indexes the associated construct(s). To repeat this important point: The measures taken in an experiment represent more than the variables; they index variables as influenced by conditions.

The insidious relationship between the categories of constructs and environments can be developed further. The influence of external environment is often unspecified in BASS research, with this influence on the internal environments of the observation units unknown and unacknowledged. Often, it would appear, the environment is difficult to simulate both because of its amorphic character and because of the potential for conditions to be dynamic. The conditions of the experiment, if attended to by the observation unit, will influence the measure(s) of the treatment variable. Inconsistency in the perception of the condition likely introduces variability across observation units that may operate toward expansion or suppression or both of the treatment effect. For the most part, whether construct and environment interact and, if so, how, is unknown and infrequently examined in any phase of the experimental design. Nonetheless, intangible aspects plus the interaction of these two elements distinguish the BASS from the PS.

Because the realizations in the experiment of both constructs and environments are most often dimensional in that they both can be expressed with the qualifiers "more" or "less," likely neither can be defined cleanly. For illustrations of the difficulties with definition and their interrelationship, consider: productivity in a kinship society, genetic altruism in an enriched environment, interpersonal power in a "buyer's market," or personal fitness under crowding. As the examples illustrate, achieving satisfactory representation of both constructs and environments can present agonizing difficulties.

An implication of the generally multidimensional nature of constructs and environments for theory development is that the realizations of both are likely also multidimensional. Two translations of the implication are important to the researcher: first, the careful experimenter may choose to index conditions explicitly; and, second, measures of both variables and conditions likely should be made multivariate.

Statistics and particularly samples seem, somehow, experiment elements of a different sort in that they are more likely to be captured than either constructs or environments, because the dimensions of each likely yields a class that facilitates high quality realization within an experiment. For instance, a population can be exampled in the form of a population unit. While parameters cannot be physically exampled because there is no way to make something like a standard deviation tangible, parameters are like other common mathematical abstractions and evoke the comfort of similarity. But all theory elements are ideals and the researcher cannot avoid missing their essence(s) more or less when he brings them to realizable form. Because, at best, theory elements cannot be translated completely and purely, they should all be kept within focal consideration. Preserving the canonical form, which requires explicit consideration of all four elements, ensures that he does so.

It is interesting to note in passing that, probably because of the above reasons plus the greater assurance that one can have about populations and parameters, critiques of studies seem to focus on populations or parameters more frequently than on constructs or environments. At the same time, the more important provinces of the BASS are likely the latter.

Status of Theory Statements and Personal Theory in the BASS

We have proposed that experimental outcomes give rise to theory statements and that a theory statement is an expression on which competent researchers working within the general model will agree. Given the prior discussions about the intangible nature of constructs, including the "constructed" perception of the environment, researchers may be unwilling to accept a particular proposed theory statement posited from an experiment because they reject one or more theory-to-experiment correspondences or reject the dimensions purported in the nature-to-theory correspondences. If this occurs frequently, as we suspect it does in exploratory BASS research, the literature underpinning early topical theory may contain multiple studies but few theory statements.

When some disciplinary interest is at an early and rudimentary stage of development, there will be few proposed theory statements, and the interested scientific community may be unable to agree on the acceptance of any. The resulting personal theories are idiosyncratic, reflecting the presumptions invoked by each author. As programmatic research proceeds, the body of proposed theory statements grows and the previously rudimentary personal theories not only expand but converge.

With increasing maturity in a discipline, agreement among researchers about the topical model broadens, the number of theory statements increases and potent theory statements begin to emerge. For example, witness the increasing universality in the theory statements and the "reach" of covering theory in Zoology on the genetic constituencies of the many zoological "families." Ideally, progress in a discipline leads to a coalescence resulting in fewer but more potent theory statements. Although this progression is true for the history of many theory statements in the PS, it remains a statement of faith in the BASS.

Section II
Introduction

The liaison between Sections I and II is the null hypothesis. The domain of theory has been the focus of the first section. Our discussion so far has been unconstrained by whether it is possible to evaluate the H_0, whether such an experiment is practical. We have not explored the costs of implementing any experiment relative to the importance of the result for increasing our knowledge. Rather, we have focused on the morphology of theory as the root of the experiment that will enhance or revise it.

Section II bridges to designing and achieving experiments. On average, what can be realized is expensive. It is expensive in part because of the compromises inherent in transforming theory elements to experiment elements. But gaining access to resources and utilizing them are also always primary concerns. Sometimes adequate representation cannot be achieved no matter how generous the available resources. For example, there may an insufficient number of variables available for representing a construct. For some experiments, achieving a desired spectrum of conditions or appropriate samples may pose the most difficulties. In some cases, the most troublesome aspect may be the quality and rigor of the numerical data or, in other instances, selecting an appropriate statistical procedure. All such concerns must be addressed in various strategies for optimizing resource use and experiment yield. Section II focuses on these concerns.

The details of constructing a personal theory in the BASS embody significant differences from those found in the PS. Subsequently, the BASS suffers lack of integrating theories and even absence of efforts to integrate theory. We believe that the difficulties arise partially from inherent complexities of content, but also partially from a lack of clearly perceived process. We have wrested-out at least an initial structure detailing the painstaking route from the researcher's interesting speculation that motivates the marshalling of resources to the experiment that is "bought" by expending them. Section I was a first approximation in clarifying the inherent complexities of content; we have made explicit as much of the tacit knowledge about process as we can articulate. It is not altogether clear how much overall reduction of the complexity in theory construction faced in the BASS can be achieved, but clarifying the process certainly offers some improvement.

Even employing significant detail, the discussion of a personal theory maintains a degree of neatness because what is under examination is an ideal. Even so, as was pointed out earlier, categories tend to overlap and mix. When the move is made from personal theory to experiment, much of the clarity in the theory domain is degraded. The world of experimentation is one of necessary compromise on a variety of bases: internal processes can be captured only inexactly, theory elements interact, and subjects show variability in attention, motivation, and even in stability of criteria. These are only a few examples.

A higher degree of order can be achieved in the artificial world of the ideal than in the natural world, as the latter exhibits and even may be founded in disorder (chaos). There is promise, however, that even amid all the complexity theory development can advance in the BASS through a careful use of a structured approach. After all, the processes of implementing experiments are no more than refinements of our routine interactions with others and with nature, even though the degree of refinement may be high. The general processes of experimentation should be more comfortable than those of theory, as any presentation of experimental process is likely to reflect significant familiarities.

Perhaps most familiar, at least in works available on experimentation, are the processes concentrating on statistics and experimental design. There is no need to repeat their contents here. They are broadly available, well done, and outside our immediate focus. Neither do we treat discipline-specific issues, which clearly would be inappropriate.

Section II, which is at the core of the book, focuses on aspects of programmatic experimentation that most directly impact on the quality of theory revision. What distinguishes Section II is the meta-level treatment of experimentation that is common to all BASS. The content has a trifold organization: structuring a microcosm, capturing the effect, and explaining the microcosm—that is, design, data, and decisions.

8
Bridging From Theory to Experiment

R evision of personal theory occurs on the basis of the outcome of an empirical test. The precision of the experiment and its focus control the quality or value of the justification for the revision. The specificity with which personal theory is translated into the highest priority research hypothesis determines the precision and focus of the null hypothesis and subsequently the experimental realization. So research implementation begins in personal theory as rendered into a research hypothesis.

The Critical Role of the Research Hypothesis

Many readers may find the vigor of the above argument varies from their own experience. It may not be obvious that the critical research hypothesis necessarily has such authority or central importance. If one asks, "Is it possible for the endeavor to proceed without the research hypothesis being articulated?" the answer is, "Yes." However, every experimental outcome uses some algorithm(s) to capture the results, and the algorithm tests the tenability of some specific null hypothesis. Because that null hypothesis implicates and partially defines, or at least constrains, some research hypothesis, the unthinking experimentalist can surrender control of the research hypothesis to the algorithm. In such a case, the prospective theory statement is outside the experimenter's control and may miss the point of the motivating intent. That is, if the researcher concentrates on the choice of algorithm without serious prior formulation of a critical research hypothesis the evidence may not make the case for revising her personal theory. A common example is the use of an omnibus null hypothesis that allows a conclusion only about a significant global treatment effect when the experimenter's focal interest is the direction or magnitude or both for some specific effect(s).

When a researcher chooses an inadequate algorithm and detours around the research hypothesis as opposed to going directly through the consideration, it typically frustrates both reader and experimenter. The reader is frustrated in not gaining the insight from the study that she sought in reading the literature; the researcher's frustration is based on her having spent precious resources for a less than optimal or even a trivial return. The research hypothesis can be confronted directly by the experimenter or indirectly through the algorithm but the scientific enterprise necessitates a confrontation.

The Differing Qualities of Theory Elements

If research hypotheses are so central, why have they received short shrift in texts on design and analysis of experiments? We believe that the neglect is embedded in the nature of the BASS. Capturing the essence of a research hypothesis means, among other things, deciding on the critical characteristics of all four theory state elements: constructs, environments, parameters, and populations.

As we have examined and considered the elements of a personal theory, we find them to have disparate qualities. It seems straightforward to acknowledge that constructs and environments are at the heart of the BASS: constructs representing internal contexts and environments representing something about perceptions of external contexts. Environments are important *to the extent* that they influence internal contexts or constructs.

We understand that oftentimes environments influence constructs, but realize it is typically unclear how or by how much. Moreover, the relation is even less clear when constructs and environments are transformed to variables and conditions in any experimental implementation. Although constructs and environments are ineffable and not always independent, they are the substance of the BASS. Difficult to characterize or to capture and difficult to defend in any specific definition or realization, these elements attract our interest but play on our intellectual and scientific weaknesses.

Although all theory elements must be represented in any experiment, the quality of the experimental transforms for populations and parameters seem somehow more easily assured than the transforms for constructs and environments. Parameters and populations, therefore, are also more easily defended and, likely, more safely attacked by others than are constructs and environments. At times, there seems almost to be an implicit agreement among BASS researchers to shy away from attacking one another's less defensible realizations of constructs and environments and to do battle in the domains of experimental representations of populations and parameters.

Collegial challenges about implementations of constructs and environments are just harder to mount. Constructs are difficult to embody, environments interact with constructs in little-known ways, and the interactions are even less well understood when each theory element is transformed to an experiment element. One withholds hasty criticism of the experimental representations of another experimenter's constructs and environments when one has little assurance about her own realizations of these theory elements. When BASS researchers challenge one another, the joust most often entails the lances and maces of statistics and samples.

We have taken pains to characterize the BASS as revolving around constructs and environments and their transforms. Any discussion on these elements within a discipline-specific setting is inappropriate on our part, but a few more general observations may clarify. First, if seeking guidance in this process, the representation of constructs is broadly addressed in measurement literature and assistance may be gleaned from reading therein. Second, a research interest in construct representation lays a foundation for increasing potency of theory revision but, in and of itself, does not change personal theory. As examples consider: Does variable X have greater utility than variable Y? Is variable X a suppressor of variable Y? Is variable X valid using variable Y as a base reference? Is variable X reliable? What minimum set of variables in what combination is optimal? Answering any of these "measurement" questions may provide insight for a change in theory, but none impacts theory as directly as might occur, for example, with more thoughtful and more focused reconceptualization of the fundamental dimensionalization of the central construct.

There is more limited and less structured assistance available for the element of environments. Two helpful possibilities are likely obvious to the reader. Even with limited resources, a researcher may be able to index reports of perceptions, as a beginning for parceling-out their influence. For a significantly greater resource expenditure, one can examine environments programmatically.

Moving From
Research Hypothesis to Experiment

In the passages between theory and experimentation there are two central concerns: going from the ideal to the compromises of reality, and returning from the specific result to a generalized conclusion. One must cross the bridge from personal theory to experiment and cross again from result to theory revision. Just how potent an experiment one organizes is determined by the critical research hypothesis as captured mathematically in the prime hypothesis. However, the experiment one runs is determined by the compromises accepted in reducing the prime hypothesis to the alternate hypothesis (H_A). Let us say that differently: The value of any experiment is vested first in the potency of the critical research hypothesis, independently of whether the experiment is more or less well-designed and more or less well-run. In the final analysis, theory will be revised on the basis of the experiment that is run and for which the result is confirmed, and that actual experiment will be based on the *alternate hypothesis* and not on the critical research hypothesis as captured in the prime hypothesis. The implication is that realizing the potency of any H_P requires assured validity, achieved only through investments in design and execution throughout all aspects of the microcosm.

9
Selecting the Experiment

The number of research hypotheses to be considered as candidates for the critical research hypothesis will likely be governed by where the experimenter's personal theory is on the exploratory-confirmatory research continuum. Generally, a large number of hypotheses can be posed within exploratory research, where personal theory is not well developed. Alternatively, confirmatory research, given the researcher's specificity of intent and interest, requires only one or a select few. In either case, the principal endeavor must be to identify the hypothesis or hypotheses having the greatest impact for revising theory.

As one's personal theory moves toward the confirmatory pole of the continuum, the critical research hypothesis becomes more obvious and the experimenter's focus is directed to obtaining the empirical evidence effectively but economically. For a more rudimentary personal theory, the experimenter must also expend resources in discerning the critical research hypothesis with clarity, as well as in addressing it once framed. On average, the path toward revising theory is clearly shorter in confirmatory research for which hypotheses are more easily specified than in exploratory research.

The critical research hypothesis is the product of a unique internal process that freely varies both in how it is organized and manifested. Metaphorically, the form of the puzzle solution is the prerogative of the puzzle solver. Moreover, not only is a formal process for defining a critical research hypothesis not realizable, it is not desirable. The composition of a critical research hypothesis must be influenced by the values, interests, and ingenuity of the author. Otherwise, theory revision stagnates for want of insight and inspiration. Nevertheless, a collection of factors contribute to the internal process that results in a critical research hypothesis. Recognizing these factors leads to the formulation of strategies to assist the researcher in making decisions.

From this perspective, we present some factors that influence the processes of defining and winnowing a candidate pool of research hypotheses. Because the decision path is strictly a matter of researcher preference, we leave the construction of an exhaustive list of influences to others. We limit our discussion to the influences that impact the decision process. The first influential factors apply to the process for the researcher entertaining a single personal theory. We conclude with factors helpful in instances when the researcher is considering two or more competing theories.

Generating Candidate Research Hypotheses

At the level of particulars, the researcher must generate a set of candidate research hypotheses and settle on the most critical. We propose that this be accomplished through a two-step process. The first step will result in a set of potential theory statements, each formed of three lists. The second step will use these potential theory statements to generate the candidate research hypotheses.

Creating Lists of Candidate Research Hypotheses

We suggest that the researcher initially develop three separate lists of statements, because criteria for inclusion in each list will differ. The first list is made up of statements accepted by those who accept the topical theory of the discipline. The composition of the first list is a series of theory statements.

The second list arises from the fuzzy edges of theory. The statements in list two fail to meet the criteria for theory statements because of inadequacies in the underlying data or experimental designs. These prospective theory statements contain purported, but suspect, relations among constructs in specific populations under specified environments. Nevertheless, the constituent statements of the second list are selected for consistency with and saliency for the researcher's developing personal theory. These first two lists are derived from the literature survey.

The third list is a product of the internal world of the experimenter. It emerges from the intuition or the belief system or both of the researcher and represents the core motivation and value for conducting the experiment. The third list, to be organized as the first two into a set of statements, is developed from what the experimenter believes is inconsistent or unsatisfactory in the current state of theory. If the task can be easily accomplished, it might be useful to rank-order the second and third lists beginning with statements the experimenter considers most secure or best-founded and concluding with those he considers most conjectural.

From Lists to Research Hypotheses

Creating research hypotheses is accomplished through a variety of tactics.

1. First, consider performing both an inclusionary and an exclusionary analysis of the pool of statements for each of the three lists of candidate research hypotheses. The inclusionary analysis leads to the predictions one can make about the characteristics of the universe from the work in which the personal theory has been grounded. Parallel with this set of predictions, the exclusionary analysis identifies where potential theory statements must be verified, extended, revised, reconciled with competing theory statements, and so forth. Comparing these complementary analyses highlights any source(s) of experimenter dissatisfaction with current personal theory. At the same time, it provides a set of candidate research hypotheses out of the personal theory, incorporating the individual interests that motivate the researcher's activities.

2. An alternative way to generate hypothesis candidates is to write research hypotheses designed either to validate or invalidate the suspect information in list 2, which comprises purported but not well grounded theory statements. The purpose is to have statements in list 2 meet the criteria for list 1 or, alternatively, to alter or remove any candidate theory statement in list 2 that does not make the grade.

3. Other hypotheses can be generated by formalizing list 3 entries, which are one's own beliefs about what theory statements the anticipated experiment would generate as research hypotheses. With tactic 2 and 3, the endeavor is to examine entries from lists 2 or

3 as potential additions to list 1—that is, to include or exclude them as theory statements. These two tactics are directed at theory elements or theory statements or both. An additional tactic for generating candidate research hypotheses addresses personal theory, itself.

4. The fourth tactic is directed not at the integrity of theory elements or theory statements but at the viability of the causal model itself. As such, this tactic is at a metalevel to the others. It focuses on sharply enhancing the confidence one has in his model by putting the model itself to critical test. Consider an example: an experimenter's personal theory predicts a result that is inconsistent with topical theory. He then organizes an experiment and affirms his deductively reasoned prediction. Affirmation of the prediction markedly strengthens the experimenter's confidence in his personal theory as an explanatory system while negating topical theory, thereby forcing a paradigm shift for topical theory. By contrast, confirmation of a failure to predict requires a paradigm shift and revision of *personal* theory but is ambiguous with respect to *topical* theory. Watanabe (1960), discussed further in Chapter 16, says this is as the singular occurrence wherein a deductive process can be crucial in the creation of inductive models of explanation. It bears repeating that, if such a critical test of topical theory is undertaken, any important result varying with the theory should be confirmed independently.

Selecting the Critical Research Hypothesis

Selection of the critical research hypothesis from the lists of candidates requires that several influences be considered by the researcher.

1. An initial influence is the process of constructing a personal theory. The impact is based largely on the difficulties with (a) completing the canonical form of each theory statement and (b) sorting the bona fide theory statements from pretenders. By definition, these two refinement processes force the researcher to confront the necessity to impose or remove limitations on the generalizations that come out of a model. Wresting the details to have confidence in, the previously held beliefs that lack sufficient empirical basis for assurance, and which details are purely speculative all assist in the identification of candidate critical research hypotheses. It is clear that sharpening personal theory influences the selection of a critical research hypothe-

sis, but it is unclear exactly how that influence operates. We consider this point in detail in a later section.

2. A second and straightforward influence rises from a logical ordering of the candidates for critical research hypotheses. It is likely that evincing some candidate critical research hypotheses must precede consideration of others; for example, only if comparable stages of moral development occur in boys and girls can one examine whether the stages occur in the same order and with comparable durations in the two populations.

3. A third and also straightforward influence comes from the motivations of the researcher. One or another of the candidate research hypotheses may be more interesting or intriguing than the alternatives. The inherent interest in a hypothesis should have a large influence in the choice of the most critical. Unless evincing the critical research hypothesis holds high interest, it is likely that the process will come to a halt somewhere between the genesis of the idea and the acceptance of the final report for publication.

4. A fourth influence, refining the critical research hypothesis to its ultimate form, is like the first a "housekeeping" influence, and makes everything neat and tidy. Typically in exploratory research the personal theory elements found in a research hypothesis can be more precisely defined with the addition of supportive information. For instance, the direction of relationship between two parameters might move from being equivocal to unidirectional, given greater familiarity with data characteristics. In general, the choice of the mechanism for maximizing the precision of the critical research hypothesis is often facilitated by conducting a PILOT STUDY. The coupling of pilot studies with EXPLORATORY DATA ANALYSIS techniques (Tukey, 1977) assures rich use of limited pilot study data.

Refining the form of the critical research hypothesis, early in the development of a personal theory may be troublesome, because the elements found in the various theory statements are only generally or partially defined. This can happen when meaningful distinctions in nature may not be known, or if they are known, the basis for the meaningfulness of the distinctions may not be fully appreciated. As a result, the scope of extrapolations formed into research hypotheses from such a personal theory can be either general, because distinctions are not appreciated, or constrained, because suspected distinctions preclude a more expansive investigation. In the latter case, researchers often choose to define theory elements narrowly in the critical research hypothesis seeking to avoid suspected and potentially vitiating distinctions in nature. The implications of exploratory research for revising theory are clear: General questions lead to new, broad theory statements requiring revision to find boundaries and exceptions; focal questions lead to new theory statements requiring yet additional theory statements in order to appreciate their implications.

5. A fifth influence on the choice of a critical research hypothesis comes from the prospective contribution of alternative candidates for affecting the plausibilities of competing causal models. A means of qualifying the plausibilities of alternative critical research hypotheses comes from Bayes' (1763) theorem. One implements a Bayesian analysis by making a subjective assessment of how much each candidate personal theory, if accepted, is likely to be impacted by a critical research hypothesis. The candidate critical research hypothesis that is likely to have the greatest impact on the competition for place among personal theories is assigned highest priority. Bayes' theorem and its application are discussed in the subsequent section.

Thus far, several influences have been suggested as leading to assistive strategies for obtaining a critical research hypothesis: housekeeping to obtain the information to complete a canonical theory statement, or refining a theory element, evaluate logical influences, and assign personal value. Following is a different type of medium for developing strategy.

A Bayes' Theorem Approach to Selecting the Critical Research Hypothesis

When the researcher is interested in sorting among competing causal models, the nonempirical (i.e., mental) exercise of conducting a Bayesian analysis can winnow the field of candidate research hypotheses. The presumption here is that the researcher is not sanguine about his causal model. However, at times in the BASS, what makes a research hypothesis critical is the need to contrast alternative models competing for place. A Bayes' theorem approach assists the researcher in arriving at a research hypothesis that puts competing models to critical test.

Bayes' theorem can be employed through any of several tactics. First, the strategy: Bayes' theorem operates on a series of position statements or alternative explanations, each having some subjective probability assigned to it, with the sum of the probabilities equal to unity. For each position statement, the subjective probability represents the likelihood of that specific position statement as being the true state of affairs. On whatever basis the experimenter chooses, each of these competing probabilities is assigned prior to the experiment. Each is appropriately interpreted as the degree of belief or the plausibility the experimenter places in that specific position statement relative to each of the others. The presentation of work by Watanabe (1960), in Chapter 16, provides a justification for assigning probabilities that may have no prior quantitative basis but are necessary to the use of Bayes' theorem.

The researcher performs a mental exercise, projecting the result he believes would be obtained from the imagined experiment. On the basis of the projected result, the researcher re-examines the plausibility he now considers each competing explanation to have. He then adjusts the probabilities of some or all the position statements accordingly, retaining the restriction that the sum of the probabilities equals unity. The adjusted probabilities reflect the researcher's new understanding of the relative potencies of the purported causal models in the competition for order.

The experimenter may engage in this mental exercise for each of several possible experiments. The experiment he will choose to run, that is, the prospective critical research hypothesis he will choose to actualize, should be that prospect he believes will have the largest impact on the plausibilities he assigns to competing explanations.

The specific formulation of Bayes' theorem, in this application, is:

Given: a body of evidence and a series of causal models or explanatory schemes (S_i; $i = 1, 2, \ldots, n$) prior to an experiment;

Let: x/e/ be the body of evidence and let $p(S_i)$ be the probability that S_i (a position statement) is true.

Then: $p(S_i|x/e/)$ is the probability that S_i is true, given the evidence, x/e/; $p(x/e/|S_i)$ is the probability of getting x/e/, given that S_i is true.

$p(S_i)$ = prior probability or the plausibility of S_i before the experiment

$p(S_i|x/e/)$ = posterior probability or the plausibility of S_i, given the evidence from the experiment

$p(x/e/|S_i)$ = probability of that evidence arising if S_i is true

and Bayes' theorem is:

$$p(S_i|x/e/) = \frac{p(S_1)\, p(x/e/|S_1)}{p(S_1)\, p(x/e/|S_1) + p(S_2)\, p(x/e/|S_2) + \ldots + p(S_n)\, p(x/e/|S_n)}$$

To put the formula into words: the probability of S_1 being the true S, given the evidence, x/e/, equals the prior probability of S_1

being true times the probability of getting the evidence, x/e/, if S_1 is true, divided by the sum of the complementary terms for each S being considered. That is, the denominator is the prior probability of each S times the probability of getting the evidence, x/e/, if that S is the true S, the probabilities being summed across all candidates for S under test.

There are ambiguities in using Bayes' theorem to justify a change in the probability assigned to each position statement before and after an experiment. Chapter 16 justifies using Bayes' theorem in the face of these ambiguities through an argument that the accumulating results progressively correct any misguided assignments of probabilities to explanations.

A clinical example illustrates the general principles of Bayes' theorem as it can be used to sort competing explanations. Let's say that an examiner has determined a client is a stutterer. From a case history, the plausibility that his stutterings result from neurotransmitter imbalance is assigned a subjective probability of 0.2, that the dysfluencies result from a central nervous system (CNS) injury is assigned a subjective probability of 0.1, that stutterings are medication related is assigned a subjective probability of 0.2, that they are stress related is assigned 0.4, and that they are caused by something else, that is, none of the above, is assigned 0.1. The examiner then obtains some set of evidence, that is, runs an experiment, does a clinical assessment, or employs whatever alternative could provide appropriate evidence to support his statements. In the case of each alternative, he examines how likely it is that the obtained evidence would arise if each candidate etiology were the true state of affairs. Tanner and Birdsall (1958), among others (e.g., Green & Swets, 1966; Swets, 1964), show that the results of experiments can be entered into Bayes' theorem calculations easily if in the form of likelihood ratios.

The expression of Bayes' theorem yields the resulting probability that the considered alternative explanation is true, given the prior probabilities and the evidence from the experiment. The Bayes' theorem procedure allows the user the opportunity to evaluate change in the probability associated with each alternative statement developed from the results or evidence. To return to the earlier example, the examiner might choose to examine some alternative CNS functions if he desires to confront the probability associated with the CNS hypothesis, or, if a physician, to reduce or increase medication or to introduce meditation therapy. This last intervention might be seen to influence the behavior no matter which of the four caused it, altering every probability at the same time. Of course, that is what often comes from running a poor test on a personal theory without considering alternative explanations beforehand.

It would be short-sighted to be constrained by the example; there are many ways to employ Bayes' theorem. The more thoughtful, creative, and insightful the researcher, the more potent the alternatives he will form will be. One tactic might be to formulate as direct a test as possible, based on the integrity of each causal model; another tactic would be to formulate a set of research hypotheses that bear on one specific causal model or a subset of the considered causal models. Yet another could be to contrast alternative pairs of models as decisively as possible.

Bayes' Theorem Application Tactics

A moment of reflection reveals some potential alternative tactics to guide choice of the experiment. That is, one may opt to do a study aimed at increasing the probability of one specific personal theory without concern for the other probabilities. Alternatively, one may seek a design motivated by the desire to wipe out one personal theory by reducing its probability to zero, or be motivated to force a confrontation between two of the considered personal theories.

To give a clinical example, presume a child is being evaluated because his history suggests any of a possible hearing loss, emotional disturbance, developmental delay, neurological system impairment, or some as-yet unstated alternative causal model. In this instance, a hearing assessment is a good initial procedure to impact at least the first causal model, whereas an assessment of fine motor skills is also a good initial procedure because of its significant effect on the probabilities of the third and fourth causal models. (For additional discussion, see Schultz, 1973.)

The point is that the experiment impacts one or more probabilities, depending on what experiment one chooses to do and the potency of that experiment for each of the specific alternatives *when all alternatives are being considered simultaneously.* That last point deserves repetition: Any experiment can be judged for merit on the basis of what impact the results are likely to have on the probabilities assigned to each of the alternative causative schemes under simultaneous test.

Whatever tactic may be employed in the selection of the critical research hypothesis, the general strategy is to reduce the multifaceted ambiguities that usually cloud the emergence of mature understanding. It is these very ambiguities that force us to do more exploratory research and the progressive resolution of the questions moves us toward a single, confirmatory testing of a personal theory. The value of applying Bayes' theorem comes from the ability to determine the relative merits of a series of purported causes, that is, governing systems.

Metaphorically, what we provide here is a recipe for manipulation of probabilities. The quality and composition of the ingredients, the research hypotheses and their associated probabilities, are the prerogative and responsibility of the chef.

Arguments For and Against
Applications of Bayes' Theorem

Some statisticians reject assignment of probabilities to personal theories when the probabilities lack empirical substantiation. That is, they object to the use of any probabilities not founded empirically. Two counterarguments should be considered. First, we believe there is a rationale for the use of quantification even if it is "softer" than we would like, because this serves the longer-range goals of enhancing our understanding and theorizing. The second point, expanded in Chapter 16, is that the recurrent use of Bayes' theorem has a built-in self-correction for the probabilities assigned, resulting from the progressive accumulation of empirical evidence.

The value of using the procedure is related to the magnitude of uncertainty, that is, to the number of alternative personal theories and the relative equality of their plausibilities, in the early stage of modeling. In the face of great uncertainty, as occurs in exploratory research, a broad variety of experiments might hold high resolution value; with minimal uncertainty, as is likely in confirmatory research, only an insightfully constructed study is likely to increase one's understanding. Whether one chooses to perform a particular experiment, or any, is a decision made by balancing the potential increase in understanding against the costs of performing the study and evaluating its results. In applying Bayes' theorem, one examines alternative possible research studies and the likely outcomes from each before selecting the actual experiment to be run.

Reconsider the first clinical example. In the course of his evaluation, the clinician considers several possible explanations for a client's nonfluent speech. His choice of a next test for the client is based on the joint consideration of what possible explanations he is currently examining, the likelihood or probability of each, and what each possible test is likely to reveal. That is, the clinician chooses a test that directly impacts one or more probabilities, perhaps wiping out a tentative explanation, or sharply increasing the credibility of some alternative personal theory, or both.

Bayes' theorem analysis, by allowing contrast of the expected impact of alternative experiments on the plausibility of competing personal theories can be seen, in this way, as a relative measure of merit for deciding which experiment one wishes to run. In the same way, this form of analysis also serves as a means of evaluating the relative contribution of a line of research for removing ambiguities in one's understanding of the governing system in nature and advancing a specific causal model.

Moving to the Null Hypothesis to be Tested

No matter what the source of the critical research hypothesis, once it is written, the serial tasks are the transition from the corresponding prime hypothesis to an alternate hypothesis and then to the null hypothesis. The prior sentence is carefully worded and reflects information from Chapter 5 that merits review. The prime hypothesis is a two-stage transformation of the critical research hypothesis including all theory elements into mathematical terms. In the first of these stages, the researcher must select the dimensions to be indexed for both the construct and the environment elements of theory. The second stage is the transformation of the now-dimensionalized critical research hypothesis into mathematical form, as indexed for all four elements.

The alternate hypothesis is a compromised form of the prime hypothesis, the compromises being necessary for its realization. A prime hypothesis can be realized through many alternate hypotheses. Settling on one alternate hypothesis is often difficult. Once decided, however, the null hypothesis is determined, being the negation of the chosen alternate hypothesis.

The essence of interest in the BASS, on average, is representation of constructs and also the environments to the extent that the researcher expects these to impact the constructs. One must represent the domain of the construct as completely but frugally as possible. Representing the domain of a construct is establishing a correspondence between the information in the construct and that in the variables, with as few variables as possible while minimizing redundancy among variables. One is attempting to include all the information of the construct, with each type being represented only once and without extraneous information.

We know of no assured path through this territory, though there are polar problems to be avoided. At one pole, the experimenter should generally question a single measure representation, because, in our perception, for the most part the BASS are properly multivariate. The danger, then, in single variable representation is that one's modeling is constrained because the experiment may miss part or all of the construct, or may be biased, or whatever. Ultimately, the risk in representing constructs as single variables is doing violence to your personal theory.

Operating at the other pole, the researcher decides to measure everything in hopes of capturing the broad dimensionality of the construct. The difficulty here is that whatever useful information may be in the variable(s) is likely to be obscured by distracting information.

We propose that the reader focus on what makes sense for revision of his model. Has each prospective variable some value for being entered into the experiment? Unless the answer is a clear "Yes," he must continue to wrestle with what he believes is true about the inherent dimensionality of the construct and with how such dimensions can be opened to measurement.

10

Data Quality: The Fineness of Resolution

A ll scientific endeavor seeks universals of explanation, with the universality independent of time and place. For example, rabbits are of higher/lower intelligence than turtles here and elsewhere, now and in the future. Perhaps the greatest single assist toward universality is the reduction of phenomena from description to quantification. Numbers, by their nature, are independent of time and location and lacking in content; relationship alone is expressed.

Physical scientists quantify the external attributes of observational units, which are likely invariant. By contrast, BASS scientists quantify the outward manifestations, what might be called generally "RESPONSE BEHAVIORS," of one or more internal processes. These are probably influenced by other known and unknown internal processes all of which may vary in intensity and direction from unit to unit and in the same unit over time. Moreover, the observational units that are interesting to BASS researchers can be expected to learn and adapt as experiences accumulate.

The theory elements relating to internal processes, constructs and environments, have been examined at length in earlier chapters. They were characterized as being dimensional. Dimensionality includes being continuous rather than discontinuous and having, in general, extensibility rather than arbitrary truncation, that is—dimensionality encompasses some set of mathematical properties. Whatever representations are to be achieved in the domain of experimentation for constructs and environments must display equivalent or corresponding mathematical properties.

What we desire in the BASS is to replace qualitative description of examined phenomena with quantification. Ideally, the rules that one observes in quantifying BASS events correspond with the logic of internal processes while they are applied to observable events. Indexing observable phenomena to treat them mathematically as evidence for the tenability of a null hypothesis is referred to as SCALING.

To cite an extreme but simple example, if a researcher is interested in quantifying some attribute of houses but indexes each house by its numerical address, he would not use these "numbers" to calculate a mean. Statistical conclusion validity, in part, is based on the assurance that the scalar properties of the data conform to assumptions of the inferential algorithm. Any mismatch between data properties and algorithm requirements jeopardizes or compromises theory building.

The mechanism for considering quantification within the BASS is most often the well-known classification of four levels of measurement (nominal, ordinal, interval, and ratio scales). Historically, however, measures of behavioral phenomena in the BASS have approached but have not achieved interval scale properties. Typically, quantification of BASS events is achieved through ordinal or quasi-interval scale properties.

Psychological scaling begins with the assignment of NUMERALS to the ATTRIBUTES of something according to a set of rules. An attribute is a property of something and the attributes this discussion will address are response behaviors which by definition are observable. Initially, numerals rather than numbers are assigned because *numerals have no inherent properties* they are simply arbitrary labels or place-holders, whereas NUMBERS are open to meaningful arithmetic combination. Numbers, technically defined, are measures that combine according to the axioms of arithmetic. In the BASS, one develops measures yielding as close approximations to numbers as can be achieved. Note that the organization and development of psychological scaling adheres to the scientific tradition of trafficking only in observables—the variables—even though the focus of our interest here is in internal processes—the constructs.

Although many are familiar with the formulation of the set of scales proposed by Stevens (1951), the explicit principles for applying measurement scales are not widely known. However, a set of axioms for scaling, paralleling axiomatic development in arithmetic, has also been formulated (Reese, 1943) and these axioms clarify applications in otherwise ambiguous instances. Oftentimes, the scales of interest in the BASS are psychophysical scales and arise through re-arranging a physical scale, such as length or weight on the basis of a subject's response behavior, such as "looks longer than" or "feels heavier than." The scale does not quantify the magnitude of a process inside the subject; a scale, instead, quantifies the magnitude of an attribute of the response behavior. That is, we measure some response behavior, for example, performance on the *Porch Index of Communicative Abilities in Children* (Porch, 1974) as allowing conclusions about a construct, such as demonstrated competence for metalinguistic tasks.

Dimensionalizing Response Properties of Constructs and Environments

Reese (1943) introduces scaling by examining the underlying internal processes, the most basic of these DISCRIMINATION: A is discriminably different from B. All nonphysical measurement is based in an ability to perceive some difference between two objects or events. The stage following discrimination is CATEGORIZATION. To categorize things as *alike* is to establish equality in some attribute and thereby to overlook discriminable differences. In this sense, discrimination results from a sensory process of being able to discern differences, whereas categorization is a symbolic or labeling system of ignoring differences to assign equality. The underpinnings of discrimination and categorization are fractioned-out in an axiomatic presentation of scaling.

The Axioms of Scaling

The initial step in Reese's axiomatic presentation is to define a single logical operator signifying discrimination. The operator: $>$, means "more of some quality in what precedes the operator than in what follows it." Examples include prettier, more severely aphasic, more cultured, more highly structured, more evolved, smarter. The operator ($>$) defines the discrimination procedure that is the foundation of all measurement, as measurement proceeds from discrimination.

Discrimination affords a nonidentity response: A ≠ B. Categorization requires discrimination. Having established categories, one can then enumerate or count members and thereby, for the first time, apply some kind of numerals. In Steven's (1951) terms, the combination of discrimination and categorization alone gives rise to a NOMINAL scale, which requires only that different attributes be categorized separately and labeled differently. Reese (1943) requires more than this for any scale but, for many purposes, the inclusion by Stevens (1951) of a nominal scale has utility and should be maintained.

The scaling of an attribute is appropriate only when one deals with nondichotomous attributes. All observation units or events have attributes. Some attributes are dichotomous-present or not present but not present in a greater-than or lesser-than magnitude. Others are present in a greater or lesser magnitude and, thereby, dimensional; being dimensional, they can be scaled.

Scaling of attributes is a stage beyond counting so that one can count anything that can be scaled. However, because scaling can occur only for attributes that can be dimensionalized, the researcher cannot necessarily scale anything she can count.

Dimensions are of two types: INTENSIVE and EXTENSIVE. The requirements of an extensive dimension subsume all those of an intensive dimension, as will be seen in the axiomatic presentation that follows. Because the operator (>) can be used to rank order examples of an attribute, for example, "feels slipperier than," an intensive dimension can yield an ORDINAL or RANK ORDER scale. Observation units demonstrating attributes on an intensive dimension cannot be combined (as is already known about specimens in a rank-order scale).

To summarize this introduction to scaling, scaling in the BASS does not lead to a quantification of anything inside the human being. That is, scaling is not a quantification of a construct; rather it is quantification of the outward manifestation of the construct measured as a variable. To assure interobserver reliability and common definition, scaling is constrained to quantifying response behaviors. As examples, one does not scale intelligence, she scales performance on the Wechsler, one does not scale pathology from the presence of vocal nodules, she scales perceived breathiness; one does not scale rage, she scales specifically defined, observable manifestations of interpersonal violence. The basis of measurement requires that there be some quantifiable behavioral attribute such that observation units can demonstrate the variable being scaled to a greater or lesser degree.

Science requires the creation of general principles from the observation of phenomena, classifying them to catch their commonalities—their essences—and extracting general patterns. First, the phenomena must be characterized as either having or lacking the same essential properties, that is, finding equalities or distinctions. However, only special sorts of equalities or distinctions are of the essence. In fruits, one can and will ignore the differences between osage oranges and navel oranges or between Florida juice oranges and Israeli juice oranges to capture the essential identity shared by all of being oranges. That is, initially one must be able to measure distinguishing characteristics, then she must decide which are nonessential for capturing essences. In this sense, scaling is only a special case of the general process of observing nature and extracting the essences of each of the elements for the building of theory.

The axioms of scaling are applied serially and each presumes all prior axioms. The number of axioms whose conditions can be fulfilled determines the scalar level of the data.

The three underlying psychological processes in scaling are discriminating, establishing equality, and categorizing. This level of scaling establishes an INTENSIVE DIMENSION and thereby an ordinal scale. Achieving it requires that the following seven axiomatic conditions be met:

Axiom I. If $A > B$, then $B \not> A$.

If A has some relation to B, for example, more debilitating than, then B cannot have that same relation to A.

The first axiom establishes ASYMMETRY in responses on the same dimension, for example, more or less careful enunciation, as specimens are ordered by the operator ($>$) in only one direction. The next axiom establishes TRANSITIVITY by carrying the asymmetry from observational unit to observational unit.

Axiom II. If $A > B$ and $B > C$, then $A > C$.

Consider as an example of Axiom II that, if A is judged to have poorer intelligibility than B and B is judged to have poorer intelligibility than C, then A will be judged to have poorer intelligibility than C. In this instance, the response behavior meets the criterion of transitivity.

The next three axioms establish the EQUALITY that is necessary if observational units are to be placed in the same category. Given that the responder sensory system operates as a discriminator rather than as an equalizer, equality is determined only indirectly and requires three axioms or sets of conditions to be achieved.

To illustrate the relation among Axioms III, IV, and V, consider an example on the perception of tonal pulses. The example gradually unfolds through the discussions of Axioms III–V. The reader is reminded that around 1000 hertz (Hz), a difference of 3 Hz or less is nondiscriminable by human beings, but greater differences can typically be perceived. Let A be the response to the perception of 1002 Hz, B be the response to the perception of 1000 Hz, and C be the response to 998 Hz tonal pulses.

Axiom III. A $\not>$ B and B $\not>$ A.

Axiom III states that A is NOT "something discriminably different" from B, for example, taller than, and B is the same NOT "something discriminably different" from A. Returning to the example, the criteria of Axiom III are met because A is not different from B, as the tones are not discriminably different.

Axiom IV. If and only if A > C, then B > C.

In this case, the pitch of A is heard as higher than the pitch of C. Response A differs from that of C, whereas the B response is not different from C. Thus the difference in responses violates the equality necessary for meeting the axiomatic condition.

Axiom V. If and only if A < C, then B < C.

Given the violation of Axiom IV in the prior example, had axiom V been tested, response A would have revealed not only that the tone triggering A was not lower than the tone triggering response C, but higher. By contrast, the tone triggering response B is indiscriminable from that triggering C, and therefore axiom V is also violated. Had A been the response to 1001 Hz, B remained the same, and C been the response to 999 Hz, a state of equality would have been established, as all three axiomatic conditions would have been met.

Axioms III to V establish equality for individual objects but are not sufficient for establishing basic DIMENSIONALITY and therefore scalability of attributes. Achieving dimensionality requires *asymmetry, transitivity, equality*, and also requires meeting the criteria of the *transitivity of the equality* and the *symmetry of the equality*, necessitating Axioms VI and VII, respectively.

Axiom VI. If A = B and B = C, then A = C.

If A is judged as being as hearing handicapped as B and if B is judged as being as hearing handicapped as C, then A must be judged as being as hearing handicapped as C.

Axiom VII. If A = B = C, then C = B = A.

Axiom VII holds that the ordering cannot be influential. As a counter-example in which ordering is influential, consider a case with a person estimating weights by picking up stones. Two stones appear equally heavy when she picks up stone 1 prior to stone 2, because 2 actually weighs less but she has fatigued herself a bit in picking 1 up first. In such a situation, the stones will not appear equally heavy if she picks up stone 2 first.

When these seven axioms are found to hold, the attribute being examined is *dimensional* on an intensive dimension, and one can construct an ORDINAL or RANK ORDER scale. Likely it is generally known that most attributes of interest in the BASS are scalable at the ordinal level. To achieve an interval level of scaling, however, requires the ability to combine observational units within the dimension and that one can estimate relative spacing between categories.

Both activities, being able to combine observational units and being able to determine the relative spacing, require the property of ADDITIVITY, and additivity is the key to an EXTENSIVE DIMENSION. Additivity is arrived at by meeting the condition of Axiom VIII. But, as will be seen, Reese (1943) presents three additional axioms to clarify possible ambiguities and to achieve a true interval scale.

Axiom VIII. If A = A' and B > 0, then A + B > A'.

For Axiom VIII to hold for intelligence, for example, one would have to be able to combine the response behavior reflecting intelligence of an individual with an IQ score of 100 with the response behavior reflecting intelligence of someone measuring 50 in IQ score so as to have greater combined response behaviors reflecting intelligence than that of another person, who also has a measured IQ of 100.

As a counterexample, suppose vitamin E were found to add some constant amount of intelligence to anyone consuming a specified daily dose—though how one could find such a result is unclear. If this were so, one could use this marginal gain, being that it is a constant, to make an interval scale of IQ. The procedure would be to take someone from any category, for example, IQ equal to 100, feed this person vitamin E, and then remeasure the individual to see what the increment was when added to the category 100. If it were discovered that the added IQ was 9, so that a person with IQ of 100 when taking vitamin E, scored equivalently to someone with IQ of 109 who was not taking added vitamin E, one would declare the vitamin E supplement to be worth 9 IQ points. Of course, because IQ is only a rank-order scale, the same vitamin E might have moved another individual from 90 IQ to 103 IQ, making the increment appear to be 13 points, or moved someone from 125 to 128, making the increment appear to be three points, or—but that is the essence of one problem with a rank-order scale.

If the addition of vitamin E to someone with IQ of 50 moved her to identity with someone of 70 IQ, then the former 70 would now have to be labeled as 59 or, alternatively, the 50 would have to be relabeled as 61. Likewise, if someone with a measured IQ of 140, on taking vitamin E scored identically with a nondrug-taking person having a score of 143, then 143 would have to be relabeled as 149. That is, using vitamin E with a large number of persons of different nondrug IQs, the steps between categories can be adjusted so that they are all equal and all categories would then be relabeled for consistency. In this manner, given the constant increment added by doses of vitamin E, an additive scale for measured intelligence could be achieved.

As the reader is aware, the construct in one person cannot be added to the construct in another, and the manifestations, that is, the variables, cannot be added either. For the internal processes that are the focus of the BASS, one cannot get to additive scales. By contrast, for the most part, sensory systems, that is, processes at the interface of the external and internal worlds, may yield higher level scales.

For any attribute to have the property of extensiveness, it must be additive. For example, one can place two sticks end to end and have the equivalent of a longer stick. That is, one can achieve additivity in length, given that length is the single characteristic being examined, all other attributes of sticks being ignored. By contrast, one cannot combine half a bucketful of water at 40° F or C with half a bucketful of water at 50° to obtain a bucketful of water at 90°; the volume of water has additivity, the temperature does not.

Axiom IX. If A + B = C, then B + A = C.

Axiom IX requires that the order in which the addition is done make no difference. In combining the shorter sticks to achieve a greater length, it cannot matter whether stick A is butted to the right or left end of stick B.

Axiom X. If A = A′ and B = B′, then A + B = A′ + B′.

That is, it cannot matter which specific observational units from a group of observational units with presumably equal magnitudes of the attribute are chosen for combining; equivalent combinations must retain equality.

As a reminder, all observation units that are measured as having the same value are defined as equal. To illustrate Axiom X, return to a presumption that intelligence as a construct has additivity, which we know it does not and cannot have. For the example, everyone with an IQ score equal to 100 is defined as being of equal intelligence in whatever study led to the construct being realized through the variable of IQ. If N persons were chosen from IQ score category A (IQ = 100) and M persons were chosen from category B (IQ = 120), and an observation unit for each of A and B were combined in each of two A+B pairs, then the performance of the combinations would also be equal, no matter which A representative combined with whichever B representative.

Axiom XI. If (A + B) + X = C, then A + (B + X) = C.

Axiom XI requires that the order of combining cannot matter. By contrast, combining order does matter in mixing cake batter and in water–acid combinations.

Once again, when examination ensures that the attribute under appraisal conforms to all 11 axioms, the scale has INTERVAL properties, also called equal-interval or equal-appearing-interval. The final axiom introduces a zero, and allows use of a RATIO scale. That is, Axiom XII completes the requirements for using *numbers*, allowing manipulation by the remaining arithmetic basic operators (x, ÷).

Axiom XII. If A = A′ and B = 0, then A + B = A′.

Commentary

Stevens' (1951) discussion, which is relatively broadly known, is well cast and helpful in considering applications of various forms of quantification. For some measurement circumstances, the Stevens' discussion is sometimes insufficiently detailed to help resolve ambiguities and uncertainty in justifying selection between data-combining procedures. For those instances with a question about which scale level the data may be at, rigorous application of Reese's (1943) axioms should resolve ambiguities.

Revision of theory is driven by empirical evidence. One seeks to maximize the correspondences between the qualities of the derived measures, the variables, and the qualities of the constructs required for better explanatory schemes. Often evidence is obtained using variables chosen in earlier studies by others without examination of their applicability to the new study. The precision offered by this axiomatic development may assist in determining what level of data (e.g., nominal versus ordinal versus [quasi-]interval) an experiment generates and thereby also assist in determining the appropriate relations between and among data sets in the path to articulating theory. That is, construction of theory is possible using any hierarchical level of measures when selected and applied carefully, because the presence and use of any coherent set of combining rules in and of itself asserts an underlying governing system or theory.

In many loci within the BASS, there appears to be a view that if researchers are careful, insightful, and lucky, they can capture data that have interval properties and, eventually, ratio properties. In addition, BASS researchers routinely treat many data as meeting the requirements for interval data. Because, most often, constructs of interest to the BASS that can be captured only through external manifestations are internal events, Reese's axiomatic presentation makes apparent that measurement mostly stops with Axiom VII and additivity cannot be achieved.

Given little reason to conclude that the BASS are predicated on constructs leading to interval or ratio scalability of variables, it is generally misdirected for an experimenter to struggle in hope of finding dimensions offering additivity. Certainly one can borrow PS constructs such as time or distance, many of which tend to be attributes of observable entities, so that interval or ratio scaling properties may be achieved for these variables. However, it is not possible to achieve the same scaling processes in representing internal processes. Trying for interval or ratio data when the basic process is without the necessary dimensionality is nonsensical. Rather, the more salient goal for the BASS researcher is to seek to capture the multidimensionality of constructs and environments through complete but frugal sets of variables and conditions at whatever scalar levels are indicated.

Examining the axioms does more than illuminate the differences between the BASS and the PS. Yet frequently, it seems that the struggle has been to make the BASS like the PS. Recognizing the essential differences between these two categories of science clarifies the unique character, purpose, and challenge of BASS theory.

11

Integrity of Data and of Parameter Estimators

At long last, having expended considerable resources determining one's personal theory and the critical research hypothesis, transforming constructs to variables to obtain the null hypothesis to be tested and then designing, implementing, and conducting a valid experiment, the experimenter finally has some data. His most modest of expectations should be that the data allow comment on the critical issue(s) rather than only on some statistical artifact. Frequently, texts in experimental design and statistics abridge any discussion of the steps in mapping the empirical data onto the alteration(s) of personal theory that they imply.

By contrast, we consider the stage of data examination prior to application of inferential algorithms to be important for two reasons. First, early and "hands-on" manipulation of the data provides the researcher with a richer sense of them than he gets from only energizing a computerized application of some statistical algorithm. Because one's motivation is to make the most powerful statement about theory that the results will allow, immersing oneself in the sample data is desirable and probably necessary. The second reason is the obvious need for assurances about the quality and consistency of data. Definite steps can be taken in early data analysis that assist in providing the appropriate security. We will deal first with the latter reason, the quality of the data.

The Quality of Data

Data integrity is assured through an examination of statistical conclusion validity. The primary concern is that the product of the inferential algorithm is trustworthy regarding the tenability of the null hypothesis. That assurance is rendered by establishing that: (1) the numbers submitted to the inferential algorithm represent what is purported for them; and (2) the application of the algorithm is statistically legitimate.

Raw Scores and Derived Scores

At the conclusion of data collection, the data often exist in some raw form. Frequently, these must be transformed to a set of derived scores prior to applying an inferential algorithm. Consider these common examples of raw score to derived score transformations: 180 responses on the *Porch Index of Communicative Abilities* (PICA) (Porch, 1981) are transformed to 18 subtest means which, in turn, are converted to three modality and one overall percentile scores; a collection of magnitude-estimation scaling scores is submitted to a log transform; air-conducted auditory thresholds at 0.5, 1.0, and 2.0 KHz are averaged to derive a single descriptor of hearing sensitivity.

In the BASS, the unit of analysis may or may not be the unit of original measure. It is important to recognize that the preliminary examination of data integrity must begin with the raw scores. Return for a moment to the PICA scoring example. Let us propose that a data recording error occurred on subtest A. If that single erroneous data point is left uncaught, two units of analysis—the graphic modality percentile and the overall percentile—will be contaminated.

Our example is not an indictment of failure of some fictitious researcher to comprehend correct application of the PICA scoring protocol. Our working assumption is that we are all competent researchers, but that nothing more than human nature mandates eternal vigilance. Opportunities for inadvertent data contamination are ubiquitous within the research enterprise: the coding of observation decisions; field recording of data point; re-recording of data points to some master file; transformation of raw to derived scores; and the transfer of data to electronic form.

None of us likes to dwell on and some may desire to reject the notion of fallibility. This seeming need for faith-in-self is undermined by the universal human failing, occurring from time to time in each of us, to make errors while completing tasks, mundane, important, or both. The classic example from the physical sciences is that of the meteorologist who, momentarily distracted during a routine task, inadvertently records an air temperature in degrees F when all other data points are recorded in degrees C. An example in communication disorders is the occurrence of an addition or division error in calculating a pure-tone average or a miscalculation of PICA subtest scores. The more likely that one responds to such examples as not being applicable to self, the more at-risk one may be for error in all stages of data manipulation.

The first level of the preliminary data examination, then, is no more but no less than double-checking and proofreading. Moreover, it is essential that this process be applied to the raw scores and again to the derived scores. While this endeavor is far from exciting, it is necessary to support a systematic evaluation of statistical conclusion validity.

Examining Outliers and Potentially Contaminated Data

We emphasize the mundane environment in which many human errors occur at the risk of characterizing the errors as trivial. To the contrary, the concern here is to eliminate erroneous INFLUENTIAL DATA POINTS. An influential data point is one that causes the interpretation of the inferential algorithm result to be biased. That is, when the influential data point is removed from the data set, the interpretation of the regression equation or the interpretation of the discriminant function, or whatever, changes as well. Once such a data point has been identified, establishing its (in)validity is of primary importance.

Fortunately, statisticians have given us a variety of tools to identify suspect data points. The clean-up techniques and the data on which they operate have been discussed under different titles, and, at the risk of some minimal redundancy, we discuss some of these tools. However, there are sharply different views about how and when, if ever, it is appropriate to manipulate experimental data prior to applying an inferential algorithm.

Regardless of whether suspect data points are legitimate or influential, they are all in some manner different from the remaining body of data. Barnett and Lewis (1984) use the term CONTAMINANT to describe a data point that, for whatever reason, represents other than what the investigator intended for it to represent. A contaminant might result from human error, technical error, an experimentally correct observation of a special but unanticipated subset of the target population, or from the proper but unintended observation of a member of some population other than the target population. Contaminants may or may not be readily discernible. Only when the value is noticeably different from the remaining data points can the contaminant be identified by value alone. For example, an observation from a second and unintended population that converts to a sample-based z score of $+1.15$, but is actually a contaminant, may very well go undetected. If this single contaminant were to be undetected, it would probably have a negligible impact on the interpretation of the analysis. But suppose the contaminant converted to a sample-based z score of $+3.25$. Such a data point might very well influence the interpretation in a small set of data.

Most often, influential data points are extreme scores. An EXTREME SCORE is one or a set of scores that take on either the greatest or least value in the collection of sample data (Barnett & Lewis, 1984). Note that every data set has extreme scores and that the extreme scores may cluster very closely with the remainder of the data points. As a result, extreme scores may or may not be influential and may or may not be contaminants.

An observation that turns out to be an extreme score and noticeably distanced from the reminder of the scores is called an OUTLIER (Barnett & Lewis, 1984). Outliers are always extreme scores, but they may or may not be valid data. According to Barnett and Lewis (1984), an outlier is "an observation (or a subset of observations) which appears to be inconsistent with the remainder of that set of data" (p. 4).

Ensuring data quality hinges on removing all contaminants, while retaining all valid scores whether extreme or not. To remain with our example, the reader is reminded that a normal distribution and random sampling will occasionally yield a data point that converts to a sample-based, or a population-based, z score of $+3.25$. While such a valid observation is not likely, superior experimental rigor and sampling theory allow it as a possibility. Nevertheless, the search for contaminants most likely begins with examination of outliers.

Empirical Data Diagnostics

Extreme values departing radically from the remaining data points can be identified solely on the basis of an inspection. An examination of z scores assists. However, the meaningfulness of the distance separating an extreme score from the rest of the data set is not always clear. For this reason, statisticians have developed analysis tools to help identify outliers. A definitive description of these tools, termed DISCORDANCY TESTS, can be found in Barnett and Lewis (1984).

Identification of a contaminant employs a different decision base than that used for identifying an outlier. Decisions regarding contamination in a data set must be made on any of a variety of bases, including intuition, clinical insight, observation-unit history, subject interviews, integrity of the original records, and re-examination of the data collection process. The point is that finding contaminants involves considerations other than the data points themselves; interpretation can come only from the experimenter's knowledge of the topic.

Decisions Regarding Problematic Data

Deciding the most appropriate response to the presence of problematic data points is a difficult step in the process of maximizing statistical conclusion validity. If it can be determined that the contaminant is nothing more than an alteration of a valid observation through some correctable human error, the course of action is clear and simple. However, if the contaminant is the product of human or technical failure that is not correctable, the data point must be discarded and possibly replaced.

The response alternatives are much different when the prospective contaminant is found to be a valid observation of a unit that is qualitatively different from the remainder of the population in some meaningful way. Such an occurrence might result from the valid observation of some previously unidentified portion of the target population, revealing that the experimenter's personal theory is incomplete and needs revision. Of course, the form of that revision will probably not be clear on the basis of one or a few observations in a data set intended for another purpose. The researcher will certainly wish to acknowledge the saliency of the suspect data points.

Further, the researcher may decide to dismiss these data points from the originally intended analysis and to study the subgroup separately. Observing additional members of the subpopulation should occur in the current or in a subsequent study. In either case, the researcher's model expands appropriately to include the newly identified complexity.

When a contaminant can be attributed to the observation of a member of a second and unintended population, the researcher must decide if the second population should be incorporated into personal theory or if the observation is nothing more than a nuisance. Where the second population represents a meaningful real world sophistication of the model, then a separate analysis and a revision of theory as described above may be indicated. Otherwise, the observation can likely be discarded. It needs to be noted that not all statisticians subscribe to the notion of discarding data points.

Accommodating Through Robust Statistics

Barnett and Lewis (1984) describe a variety of techniques to evaluate the tenability of a null hypothesis based on a data set containing one or more outliers. They term the application of such techniques as an ACCOMMODATION STRATEGY. The recommended techniques are resistant to the negative effects of outliers, so that, in Barnett and Lewis's terminology, the strategies accommodate outliers. Statisticians refer to this family of inferential algorithms among others as ROBUST STATISTICS. The Type I error rate of a robust statistic remains at the nominal level regardless of the presence of outliers. Other robust statistics accommodate population distribution characteristics that would contraindicate more well known algorithms.

Robust statistics, then, are alternatives to traditional inferential algorithms. When the assumptions of traditional algorithms cannot be met, the statistical conclusion validity of an analysis is compromised, whereas use of analysis based on robust statistics is not.

Implications of Choice of Strategy for Theory

Unfortunately, there is no simple set of rules for choosing among these strategies or even any clear, universal principles to guide the decision process. The researcher must find what guidance he can from consideration of the importance of the exceptional data to his own interpretation and, consequently, to the model under focus. That is, decisions about whether to separate out the atypical data or to accommodate them are based in the personal theory or the interpretation the researcher chooses to put on the study.

Should data, for example, suggest that the personal theory may apply differently to a second, previously unsuspected population, the researcher can stop to consider whether such sophistication is in his focus of interest at the time. Deciding "Yes," he can specifically examine the atypical data, generate a new study with subjects chosen from the newly perceived population, or some alternative tactic directed at this variant.

Decisions about focusing on valid atypical data represent some amount of shifting in the focus of one's sophistication and personal theory. Should the experimenter determine he is interested in the more typical data, he must decide whether to retain the atypical data in the analysis or set them aside in the analysis, and comment on them in text. The principle that theory building, as a progressive sophistication of personal theory, is best served by attending to all valid data is the appropriate guide for the long-term goals of science. The responsible experimenter does not ignore or fail to report valid, structured observations of nature.

Advancing the Data Analysis

Calculation of derived scores begins once the researcher is satisfied that the raw-score data set has been cleaned up. Since the calculation of derived scores represents an opportunity for injecting error, we recommend that these calculations be conducted through a computer program. Moreover, we recommend that the raw scores be transferred to electronic form early and that the preliminary data analysis be conducted on the electronic data set.

When derived scores become the units of analysis, the secondary set also must be examined for a valid application of an inferential algorithm based on tenability of the assumptions about the parent population. Achieving maximal statistical conclusion validity may call for a nonparametric statistic, such as FRIEDMAN'S F or WILCOXON'S MATCHED PAIRS, or a modified statistic such as Windsorized means, or a robust statistic like C, depending upon the nature of the data structure.

The Characteristics of Data

Coming to understand the richness of the data set, especially in early stages of paradigm development, is likely facilitated by use of Tukey's (1977) *exploratory data analysis* (EDA). This is equally true for raw and derived scores. EDA techniques, such as STEM AND LEAF displays and BOX-WHISKER PLOTS are particularly useful for exploring, understanding, and summarizing data. Note that, unlike exploration of contaminating or outlier data, the emphasis at this stage of analysis is primarily the sample and not the population. The interested reader is referred to Tukey's elaborated presentation on the topic.

Often the greatest insight into the structure of a data set is obtained by plotting various quantities. For example, the best way to determine if the data in a two-way analysis of variance are characterized by an ORDINAL, wherein the patterns are not parallel but do not intersect, or a DISORDINAL interaction, with the patterns intersecting one another, is to plot the cell means. Tukey (1977) advises data explorers to make generous use of graph paper, tracing paper and pencils—plotting and replotting data in almost every way one can conceive. We heartily agree.

Of course, calculation of the usual descriptive statistics is routinely indicated. MEANS, MEDIANS, VARIANCES, PROPORTIONS, CORRELATIONS, and so forth are at the heart of the interpretations coming from any analysis. We would note that, in the BASS literature, presentation and interpretation of DESCRIPTIVE STATISTICS are often completely limited to the sample. While it is true that descriptive statistics characterize only the sample, they are also, by definition, estimates of population values. As such they play an important role in the expansion of personal theory. A researcher cannot accept any point estimate blindly and hope to revise theory insightfully.

Ensuring High Quality in Parameter Estimation

Integrity of a new statement of theory on the basis of a parameter estimate, which is the product of applying some algorithm, is dependent on three mathematical properties associated with the ESTIMATOR or algorithm. Hopkins and Glass (1984) term these properties: UNBIASEDNESS, EFFICIENCY, and CONSISTENCY.

Unbiasedness, efficiency, and consistency are all characteristics of the sampling distribution of an estimator. A point estimator is unbiased when the mean of its estimates equals the population value. When this is not the case, the estimator is said to be negatively or positively biased. Fortunately, many common estimators, for instance, variance, have been shown to be unbiased.

According to Hopkins and Glass (1978), the *efficiency* of an estimator is an issue of precision across samples. The index of efficiency is the magnitude of the STANDARD ERROR of the sampling distribution. Because the standard error decreases as the sampling error decreases, so estimator efficiency increases as the standard error decreases. The relative efficiencies of two competing estimators are given by a direct comparison of their standard errors.

Unbiasedness and efficiency are measures on the sampling distribution of an estimator for a particular sample size. By contrast, estimator *consistency* arises from the sampling distributions for an estimator across many sample sizes. A point estimator is consistent when the estimation of the parameter improves as the sample size increases.

When a researcher intends to build theory through parameter estimation, careful consideration of the mathematical properties of the point estimators is indicated. The unbiasedness, efficiency, and consistency of the estimator will govern the quality or trustworthiness of the parameter estimate. Moreover, the product of a satisfactory estimator should not be taken as a dead reckoning. Rather, the precision of the estimate should be qualified by a confidence interval. Further, the researcher should take care to build one-sided confidence intervals to complement one-tailed null hypotheses. While the general practice of building confidence intervals is particularly valuable for the purpose of theory building, it is often neglected in BASS literature.

In summary, parameter estimation is an underrated aspect of systematic theory building. Careful parameter estimation requires consideration of estimator precision, to be undertaken at the level of the estimator and also at the level of the estimate.

Evaluating the Tenability of the Null Hypothesis

At this point, the preliminary data examination process comes to a close. The next step is to submit the data to the inferential algorithm of choice. The researcher now examines all the validities for his first-choice inferential algorithm to decide whether its assumptions are tenable given the obtained results. If the sample-based information contraindicates application of that algorithm, he can entertain an alternative. But a researcher with data must settle on some inferential algorithm that is valid in retaining tenability when considered against the various validities for revision of personal theory. Moreover, his principal consideration is that he not sacrifice potency to arrive at a valid algorithm. There are classes of algorithms available to the researcher, with the distinctions between the classes in the underlying assumptions. Because of the available variety, the researcher should be able to select an algorithm with assumptions that can be met, so that he need not consider alteration of his statistical hypotheses. Choosing an algorithm is the subject of the next chapter.

The calculations are best carried out by a computer-based statistical computation package (for authoritative assistance, see all volumes of Barcikowski, 1983). Whatever program one might choose, we recommend that calculations be done on two separate packages. This suggestion is based on the fact that different packages have different default operating assumptions (e.g., WEIGHTED versus UNWEIGHTED MEANS, two-tailed versus one-tailed tests). When identical results are obtained from two different packages, the results can be interpreted with confidence.

Having completed the processes described in this and earlier chapters, a researcher will be in a position to make two requisite decisions in a straightforward fashion. The first is whether to reject or fail-to-reject the null hypothesis. The basis for the second decision is whether the results are meaningful or trivial. The evidence for this latter decision is given by the a priori definition of meaningfulness. What remains, then, is to explain why the results turned out as they did. Other things being equal, the elements of this explanation are the products of the preliminary data analysis (e.g., plots and descriptive statistics).

Whatever the outcome, the results will maximally comment on the critical research question and minimally comment on artifact issues. That is, the statistical conclusion validity of the study will be maximized and, as a result, the ability to revise theory on the basis of the study will also be maximized.

12

Choosing Among Statistical Tests

Consistent design and construction of routinely high-quality experiments requires knowledge and mastery of a broad range of skills. Some, such as selecting important problems or selecting critical parameters reflect mastery of conceptual insights as well as sensitivity to the patterning of natural events. These are at the heart of important research and represent the connoisseurship of a discipline. Other expertise, such as implementing an experimental design or conducting a numeric analysis is more technical or more easily defined and structured and, therefore, can be subject to criteria of successful mastery. Determining the statistical-test-of-choice for an experiment is found between these extremes. Making a high quality choice involves aspects of connoisseurship but also entails mastery of technical skills. This chapter is designed to provide as much structure as we can extract for this often troublesome step in the empirical process.

The key to the structure is that inferential algorithms map onto null hypotheses. Valid and potent null hypotheses and their preceding alternate hypotheses can only come from potent prime hypotheses.

Like much of experimental implementation, choosing a statistical test is a task of optimizing across a series of compromises. Further, statisticians do not share uniform views about the efficacies of different statistical tests or classes of tests. Because of such differences, the general rules presented in this chapter must be viewed as somewhat arbitrary and arguable. There are no standard procedures or solutions for almost any class of experiments and, often, even the range of options is not apparent. An experimenter hopes to zero-in on a statistical-test-of-choice to maximize the correspondence between the prime hypothesis and the quantification of the observed effect through application of an algorithm. Further, one wishes to avoid having a less than thoughtful choice of algorithm determine the tested null hypothesis.

By way of reminder, the hypothesis of interest is the prime hypothesis. The prime hypothesis is the mathematical translation of the critical research hypothesis, which is the product of some proposed causative model, and the alternate hypothesis is a realizable best approximation of the prime hypothesis. The null hypothesis is then formed as the exclusive and exhaustive counter hypothesis, the negation of H_A. But the H_A can take on multiple forms and more than one can be potent. The relative appropriateness of each has to be estimated by some sort of a cost/benefit payoff matrix plus the interests of the experimenter with respect to alternative revisions of her personal theory that the results can promote.

The choices of H_A and, therefore, of H_0 are the prerogative and responsibility of the experimenter. If the experimenter requires or feels need of assistance for choosing H_A and H_0, that assistance is better sought from a mentor than from a statistician. Such choices are best made from information and knowledge about the discipline in addition to competence in statistical procedures.

Structuring the Selection Process

Presentation of procedural modeling by detailing every statistical test and variation in experimental design is not practical. A manageable set can be achieved if we restrict the presentation to those statistical tests and designs most often reported by behavioral scientists. Largely, questions that lead to research hypotheses in the BASS involve any of the following four forms:

A. In what proportions do classes of events occur for specific populations in specific environments?
B. How do constructs relate to one another for specific populations in specific environments?

C. How do distributions of populations differ in terms of central tendency for specific constructs within specific environments?
D. How do distributions of populations differ in terms of variability for specific constructs within specific environments?

The questions organize four obvious parameters, each comprising a family of algorithms:

A. Measures of proportion (e.g., SIGN TEST, χ^2, proportion equals a constant, proportion equals another proportion).
B. Measures of relationship (e.g., product moment correlation (ρ), C, POINT-BISERIAL CORRELATION, MULTIVARIATE REGRESSION).
C. Measures of central tendency (e.g., ANOVA, ANCOVA, MANOVA, MANCOVA).
D. Measures of variability (e.g., BOX'S M, MAUCHLY's LIKELIHOOD RATIO CRITERION, F_{max}, BARTLETT'S χ^2).

Each family encompasses a large number of algorithms. We presume the reader's knowledge of, or access to, resources for the constituency of each family in each of three classes: PARAMETRIC, DISTRIBUTION-FREE, and ROBUST STATISTICS (Marascuilo & McSweeney, 1977).

Choosing among the candidate algorithms begins with the finite set of statistical tests and winnows progressively. Determining the statistical test of choice, from this point, requires:

A. Assurance that the canonical null hypothesis has an appropriate form for the number of and choice of variables representing each construct.
B. Assurance that the canonical H_0 is directional if appropriate (one-tailed versus two-tailed).
C. Identifying the algorithm family.
D. Identifying the algorithms that map onto the null hypothesis.
E. Winnowing the pool through an iterative process by examining the mathematical properties of the estimated distributions against the assumptions to be met for use of each algorithm.
F. Winnowing the surviving algorithms on the basis of greater Type I and Type II error control. Given a choice of competing candidate statistical tests, one opts for that candidate yielding greatest value in its characteristic control of Type I (α) and Type II(β) errors.

When there appear to be equally good candidates from each of the classes of parametric, distribution-free, and robust statistics, we propose that the reader consider them ordered and go for the topmost. If at this point a statistical-test-of-choice is not apparent, consider employing a statistical consultant.

We repeat that up to the winnowing process, any consultation is for the purpose of organizing one's own thinking about the connoisseurship. For the winnowing process and beyond, a consultant assists in implementation. Likely it goes without saying that the practice of restraining research to the application of only a small pool of algorithms is not one that has effectively built and revised theory. Pursuit of critical research hypotheses requires versatility in contemporary quantification skills.

13
Optimizing for Potency in Decisions

This chapter presents a perspective on the logic of testing hypotheses. The reader is likely aware that the present form of hypothesis testing logic was conceptualized by Jerzy Neyman and Egon S. Pearson (Neyman, 1943; Neyman & Pearson, 1933) and has been articulated by many authors. Although we find utility in their general scheme, we also propose that some of the transitions from one step in the implementation process to another are neither obvious nor easily made. Therefore, we believe there is utility in recasting the steps to focus on the transitions. The more conventional Neyman–Pearson implementation, which we symbolize in text as N–P, and our adapted and expanded process are contrasted in Table 13-1. The table accentuates the contrast between a fairly common implementation of the N–P logic and our expanded procedure. Because of the implied criticism of any Neyman–Pearson presentation, no source citation is given.

The initial N–P step is to state the research problem, which is equivalent to what other authors term stating the research question. The reader is reminded that we have already introduced a helpful decision process for the steps leading up to Neyman–Pearson's first step, which are discussed in Chapters 5 and 9. We present the N–P

Table 13–1 Schemas for the Logic of Hypothesis Testing

Standard Interpretation (Neyman–Pearson Schema)	Adapted Schema
State the research question	Determine **personal theory**
State the research hypothesis	State the **critical research hypothesis**
State the statistical hypotheses	State the **critical research question**
Determine valid and reliable measures of dependent and independent variables	Dimensionalize **constructs, environments, parameters**, and **populations**
Choose a test statistic	Define the H_P
Select a level of significance	Define the variables
Decide on the power of the statistical test	Define the remaining elements
Determine the effect size	Write the H_A
Determine an appropriate sample size	Write the H_0
Determine the critical values	Operationalize all temporal and spatial contexts, all **populations** and **parameters**
Select a random sample and assign units to treatments	Choose a test statistic
	Select a level of significance
	Decide on the power of the statistical test
	Determine an effect size
	Determine an appropriate sample size
	Determine the critical values
	Effect the true or quasi-experiments

steps and our modifications for all the steps occurring prior to the gathering of data. The critical difference between our listing and conventional wisdom is the logical bridging between personal theory and experiment, giving the researcher confidence in those steps and, more importantly, in his return from experiment to personal theory.

The steps for testing hypotheses beyond creation of the personal theory can be collapsed to four criteria important to a research design. These are discussed below and embedded in the questions: (1) What makes an experiment outcome potent? (2) What constitutes compelling results? (3) What constitutes important results? and (4) How sensitive is an experiment?

The potency preserved in an experiment as a concept was introduced in Section I and is only reviewed here. The criteria of the latter three questions are emphasized in this chapter. The criterion for compelling results is established on the basis of statistical significance. The standard for importance of results is determined on the basis of what we have termed clinical significance, or the knowledge of a discipline, or the state of personal theory. The criterion for how sensitive an experiment must be is fixed in the reconciliation of the first two. To accomplish the reconciliation, one can design a potent experiment with sufficient sensitivity to evaluate clinical significance on the basis of statistical significance.

Potency of the Experiment

We earlier stated that the potency of an experiment arises from whatever prospective theory statement is chosen as the critical research hypothesis. This potency for revision of theory, first found in the critical research hypothesis, is captured maximally in the null hypothesis, given good transformations of critical research hypothesis to prime hypothesis to alternate hypothesis, and then to the null hypothesis. Once the null hypothesis is well defined, the researcher goes about the business of collecting evidence to determine its tenability. This much of the logic of testing hypotheses assures that the form of the collected evidence bears directly on the interesting question.

Convincing or Compelling Evidence

Whether or not some evidence is compelling for the decision regarding the tenability of the null hypothesis is determined by the a priori tolerance for Type I error. A typical interpretation of Type I error tolerance is that of a safeguard. A more useful definition is as a criterion for believability or for what constitutes compelling evidence. An exact probability that is less than or equal to the Type I error tolerance is convincing evidence for abandoning the null hypothesis as being tenable. For example, assume that a researcher sets Type I error tolerance at 0.05. Further, assume that the researcher determines that the exact probability for an obtained test statistic is 0.0378. The interpretation of this outcome is:

> The probability of obtaining a test size this large or larger, due strictly to chance, in a second and independent sample taken from the same population is 0.0378. Because this probability is less than 0.05, the null hypothesis is rejected (i.e., deemed untenable) in favor of the alternate hypothesis.

Readers who find this interpretation consonant with their experience may wish to move on to the next section.

The interpretation of Type I error tolerance is:

> The acceptable proportion, in this case, 0.05, of incorrect decisions in a large set of decisions, that is, in a sampling distribution, where an incorrect decision regarding a true null hypothesis is rendered solely on the basis of an atypical sample brought about by random sampling.

This interpretation is often translated to something like:

> I am willing to make a wrong decision about a true null hypothesis 5% of the time.

Although this translation is technically correct, it is not technically complete. Therefore, the translation by itself is not particularly useful for evaluating an exact probability level, because it assumes a central distribution for the statistic. In contrast, critical research hypotheses almost exclusively assume a noncentral distribution. If one is willing to entertain the possibility of a noncentral distribution, then the Type I error tolerance can be regarded as the criterion for achieving a convincing result based on the correct interpretation of an exact probability. In this sense, the Type I error tolerance is interpreted as a threshold probability beyond which an associated outcome is attributed to something other than chance alone.

Continuing with the example, the researcher in effect says:

I will conclude that something other than chance is responsible for the outcome when the magnitude of the obtained test statistic is so large that the probability of obtaining another that large or larger in a second sample is less than or equal to X. That is, I will not attribute an outcome to chance when the probability of chance being the responsible agent is less than or equal to X.

The researcher thus establishes an a priori criterion for convincing evidence. Note that when the distribution is in fact central, and all other things ideal, the researcher would come to an incorrect decision about a true null hypothesis X% of the time. If internal validity can be assured, then by deduction the something-other-than chance must be the treatment effect. The logic of this approach makes no provision for phrases like "highly significant" and "approached significance." The use of such phrases represents an ill-conceived attempt to find importance in a probability value.

Importance of the Departure
From the Null Hypothesis

Although the criterion for compelling results relative to the tenability of the null hypothesis is found in the Type I error level, the criterion for what constitutes an important departure from the null hypothesis is extracted from the test statistic. Consider the following problem: A researcher conducts a correlation analysis at $\alpha = 0.01$ and finds $r = 0.27$ with a $p = 0.0014$ for the null hypothesis: $H_0: \rho = 0$. It is clear that the inference $\rho = 0$ is not tenable; it is not clear that the departure of 0.27 from zero is an important difference. Unless the threshold magnitude for importance is stated explicitly, the importance assigned to any finding can be equivocal, even to the experimenter.

All too often, a researcher finds himself pouring over statistical results and, at that time, attempting to attach importance to the results. This practice amounts to an a posteriori or "after the fact" definition of "important findings." When one defines importance on the basis of experiment results, the sample becomes the prime entity for interpretation. Under these circumstances, any comments about the population and, therefore, about the state of one's personal theory are strictly the products of inductive reasoning, that is, the characteristics of the sample characterize the population. By contrast, a priori modeling allows application of both inductive and deductive reasoning.

A more careful application of the logic of testing hypotheses, beginning in deductive reasoning, is modeled in the following sequence:

1. A researcher hypothesizes some possible or probable quantifiable characteristic of the population on the basis of the existing personal theory;
2. The tenability of that research hypothesis is evaluated through examination of a sample drawn from the population;
3. Based on known or assumed properties of an algorithm and on previously defined error tolerances, the researcher reaches a reject or fail-to-reject decision regarding the null hypothesis;
4. The decision leads to a revision or extension of personal theory.

The relevant question is how to incorporate "important findings" into this sequence.

Rather than stating only that some characteristic exists in a population, a researcher can specify the threshold magnitude the characteristic must exceed to be considered important for theory building. Determining the minimum magnitude for a finding to be "important" can come about from any of one's own current personal theory, some other existing knowledge or clinical experience. Toward the pole of more confirmatory research, the threshold magnitude is more precisely indicated by personal theory.

Effect Size

Theory statements embody effects and critical research hypotheses do likewise. The combination of theory elements into an alternate hypothesis, in its turn, also proposes an effect. The null hypothesis negates its occurrence, so that a greater or lesser departure from the null hypothesis in a valid experiment is a measure of that effect.

In the experiment domain, the EFFECT SIZE is the magnitude of the relationship between the independent variables and the dependent variables. Treatment effects in the experiment domain correspond directly to treatment effects in the theory domain, where effect size is the magnitude of relationship of some constructs on other constructs in the context of all the theory elements. Effect size can index the *magnitude* of a relationship or the *magnitude of change* in a relationship.

Effect size in the theory domain is a parameter and is estimated as a statistic in the experiment domain. An effect size estimator is uniquely determined by the form of the associated null hypothesis, for example, the effect size estimator for a correlation null hypothesis differs from that of a frequency-of-occurrence null hypothesis. The estimators are not themselves tied to probabilities; they do not test null hypotheses but, rather, they index departures from null hypotheses.

The implication of effect size in the theory domain is discriminability. The implication of effect size in the experiment domain is sensitivity for detecting a meaningful distinction, given that one has decided that it exists in the theory domain.

To illustrate the notion of an effect size, consider the following example. Let us say that all things equal to x and y correlate at 0 from time 1 to time 2. Further, assume that previous research has shown that introducing agent A between times 1 and 2 causes $\rho = 0.7$. Suppose a researcher wishes to test a purportedly superior agent (i.e., one for which he claims greater homogenization). The researcher decides that the meaningful null hypothesis is: ρ is less than or equal to 0.7. The next question is: How large a departure from the null hypothesis is it important to detect? Is the researcher interested in rejecting the null hypothesis only if the effect size is large—that is, a large departure from ρ less than or equal to 0.7? Alternatively, is the researcher interested in detecting much smaller departures from H_0, that is, a smaller effect size? In whichever case, in rendering a decision about what constitutes an important departure from the null hypothesis, the researcher sets the quantity that the subsequent analysis must be able to detect. With that decision, he can design an experiment that is sufficiently sensitive to detect that quantity.

In this discussion, we have disregarded precise mathematical definitions for the various effect sizes and considered only the general notion common to all inferential tests. The effect size differs from the test itself, in that it has no degrees of freedom or associated error probability. It is simply a standardized, that is, scale-free, measure of departure from the null hypothesis.

The effect size in the theory domain represents an attractive index for quantifying departures from the null hypothesis to reflect the relevance of the findings for personal theory. That is, an effect size can be specified in the theory domain to serve as the threshold magnitude the obtained results must surpass to be considered important. Defining that minimum requires estimates of various parameters, and achieving satisfactory estimates prior to an experiment may be difficult. Alternatively, by following suggestions by Cohen (1988), described next, a researcher can arrive at the necessary estimates through intuition and good judgment.

Benchmark Effect Sizes.   Cohen defines small, medium, and large benchmark effect size magnitudes for each of several inferential tests, for example, χ^2, F, r, and he offers a convincing rationale for each. Cohen's benchmarks, then, represent intuitively appealing vehicles, because the math is hidden, for expressing the criterion magnitude for an effect to be important. Consider two examples. A researcher is investigating the effectiveness of a therapy for a population for which no treatment has been efficacious. In this case, any reduction of symptoms associated with exposure to treatment would be clinically useful, so even a small effect size would be important. Alternatively, let us suppose a particular reading program is used in an elementary school system, comprising some sets of workbooks, examination protocols, and so forth. A researcher compares that program with an alternative program. In this case, a large effect size would be mandated so the costs of purchasing the new materials plus those of implementing the change would have an assured substantive gain in pupils' reading skills.

The Sensitivity of an Experiment

Sensitivity in an analysis is the probability of detecting an important departure from a false null hypothesis. Therefore, achieving sensitivity requires that a researcher declare a tolerance for Type II error. Type II error is rarely reported in BASS experiments. Nevertheless, Type II error rates can be synthesized from the estimates of effect sizes found in many published reports. Literature surveys (e.g., Kroll & Chase, 1975; for additional sources, see Cohen, 1988, p. xi ff) of several BASS disciplines have found that, on average, Type II error hovers around 0.7. That is, often we may conduct experiments where, in fact, the null hypothesis is false, fail to detect the departure from the null hypothesis because statistical significance is not obtained, and conclude accordingly. Optimizing the likelihood of retaining good research hypotheses, that is, of rejecting the null hypothesis when it should be rejected, comes about through routine use of a priori power analyses.

Statistical power or $1 - \beta$ is the probability of rejecting a false null hypothesis. In his book on the topic, Cohen (1988) states that statistical power in the BASS should reach or exceed 0.8. This value is in stark contrast to the results of the previously mentioned surveys that found statistical power to be about 0.3 in BASS literature. Why does statistical power fall so low? The answer seems to be that BASS researchers typically set an a priori Type I error rate but do not specify an a priori Type II error rate, nor take steps to control it. The management of Type II error rate in an experiment requires a priori statistical power analysis.

A statistical power analysis requires three pieces of information in addition to the desired power level. These are: effect size, the Type I error rate, and the number of observation units or subjects. The four terms share a mathematical relationship so that the value of any one can be solved for, given values for the other three. As a result, it is possible to set power and Type I error at some desired levels, set the value of the effect size as indicated by personal theory, and to solve for sample size.

Given an effect size and the specification of Type I and Type II error rates, one can easily determine necessary sample size using tables provided by Cohen (1988), which are indexed by effect size, Type I error, and statistical power. The obtained sample size (n) for an effect size (x), a Type I error rate (y) and a statistical power (z) can be thought of as:

> The n necessary to detect an effect size of at least magnitude x with y Type I error tolerance at z statistical power.

Said another way, an a priori statistical power analysis yields the number of observational units or subjects necessary to detect a meaningful departure from the null hypothesis at tolerable risk levels. An a priori statistical power analysis can be thought of as an analysis of the costs of desired benefits. The cost in this equation is the number of observation units; the remaining three elements define the benefit, mostly in terms of efficiency for building theory.

Unfortunately, here as elsewhere, what one desires and what one can afford are often antagonistic. As a result, the initial power analysis is often followed by pragmatic compromise. In instances where the number of observation units necessary to conduct an unabridged experiment is excessive, one or more of the following actions is indicated:

1. Accept a higher Type I error level;
2. Accept lesser statistical power;
3. Sacrifice sensitivity of the experiment so that only a larger effect size is detectable.

Obviously, none of these actions is wholly satisfactory, because all represent less than one's best judgment. However, when compromises are necessary, the initial a priori statistical power analysis makes apparent the discrepancies between an ideal and a best-obtainable implementation. The researcher then can come to a decision across an apparent set of alternatives and make abridgments, understanding the costs in statistical conclusion validity, thereby retaining control of his analysis.

14

From Experiment to Personal Theory

Historically, the common and general understanding of the tested null hypothesis is that it yields inference only for parameters. Although this understanding is technically correct, no researcher builds theory on testable null hypothesis in canonical form, the researcher has the basis for an inferential leap about paramters on variables within the context of the other elements. That is, she is ultimately bridging from a decision about the null hypothesis to a decision regarding revision of her personal theory.

We remind the reader that bridging from the exclusive province of theory to the exclusive province of experimentation occurs in two stages. The first stage transforms dimensions of constructs to variables. If the researcher cannot do this satisfactorily, the experiment is unthinkable because no testable null hypothesis can be created. In the second stage, having selected the set of variables, she creates additional operational definitions for the remaining three elements.

The complement of the two-stage bridging from theory to experiment is that when one evaluates the tested null hypothesis for revision of personal theory, again the process is two stage. In the first stage, she must transform the experiment elements of statistics, samples, and conditions to their respective theory elements in personal theory. At this point, while she has drawn inferences about environments and populations, the parameters express variables rather than constructs. Returning wholly to theory requires the second stage of inferring to the dimensions of constructs that originally motivated the study. The quality of each inference to theory elements is ensured in its experiment validity, rather than in the probability value.

Theory revision itself may follow either of two paths. The choice of passage toward revision begins in the decision on the tenability of the null hypothesis. Conceptually, one path is taken when the null hypothesis is rejected, and the research hypothesis becomes a theory statement. The alternate path becomes her route when she fails to reject the null hypothesis and she must re-examine the status of her personal theory to discern inadequacies in her understanding. Presuming a satisfactory outcome from examination of the experiment validities on the one hand, rejection of the null hypothesis leads to a *statistical* inference on the *elaborateness* of her revision of personal theory whereas, on the other hand, failure to reject the null hypothesis leads to an *inductive* inference on the *adequacy* of her personal theory.

The Experiment Outcome Meets Expectation

One inferential leap occurs in the rejection of a null hypothesis and another occurs in the acceptance of an alternate hypothesis, with only the former based in statistical significance. That is, two inferential leaps occur in returning from the real microcosmic world of the experiment, expressed in a testable hypothesis, to the modeled world of a personal theory expressed in a research hypothesis.

We turn first to rejection of the null hypothesis, which is the inference based in statistical significance. When the exact probability (p) associated with the test size of the inferential statistic is less than the a priori Type I error tolerance (α), interpretation of the result is based in experiment validity. By way of example, say that a researcher has obtained a dependent t-statistic on 39 degrees of freedom. Assume that the associated exact p in this example is found to be 0.0066. Further, accept that the researcher specified 0.05 as the a priori Type I error tolerance level. The interpretation for the obtained value is:

> The probability of obtaining a test size this large or larger, due strictly to chance, in another independent random sample of this size is 0.0066. Because this value is below the tolerance for error due to chance, the test

size is attributed to something other than chance. Accordingly, the H_0 is rejected in favor of the H_A, pending assurances on the validities.

The something-other-than-chance explanation for the magnitude of the test size may be consistent with the research hypothesis. Obviously, this is the second inferential leap and is an attractive explanation because it embodies a valid acceptance of the alternate hypothesis. However, rival explanations for rejection of the null hypothesis are possible. These competing explanations represent threats to the validities of the experiment. When one or more of the validities suffers a serious violation, the statistical evidence may suggest that the null hypothesis should be rejected but for the wrong reason. In this case, rejection of the null hypothesis is invalid, and acceptance of the alternate hypothesis is without warrant.

In the best of circumstances, careful planning of experiments and careful data analysis rule out rival explanations. Under these conditions, the researcher concludes that the observed treatment effect is characteristic of the population(s). Because the canonical form is inclusionary, the experimenter can extend from parameters in context to inferences about the relationships of all four experiment elements and then to inferences about the relationships among theory elements. The legitimacy of each inference from experiment to theory is based in the validity of the earlier translations of personal theory to experiment. Once again the isomorphism of theory, experiment, and validity elements is apparent. The structural parallels provide a comfortable basis for interpreting the experiment's results and revising one's personal theory. That is to say, the validity or differentiated validities of an experiment provides its legitimacy for revising theory, with observance of validities monitoring the experiment.

There are limitations that *abridge the basis* of the inferential leap from an experiment. These limitations arise out of the personal theory elements. Less adequately conceptualized theory elements or inadequacies in the experiment that constrain theory revision give more limited theory. Other limitations from an experiment can *directly abridge the inference(s)*. For instance, there may be some occurrence that compromises the design; for example, the subjects in different treatment groups communicate with one another, with each group gaining information that influences performance. Alternatively, conducting the experiment reveals some previously unsuspected inadequacies that delimit the inference that can be drawn. This latter class of limitations of a study arise from the abridgments of its classes of validity or, said differently, arise from inadequacies that abridge the inference directly.

One must be assured about the *basis* of the inferential leap, given by the integrity of the transformations from personal theory to experiment elements. Chapters 5 and 13 discuss the a priori activities needed to invest inference with maximum legitimacy.

Inferences on Elements

When the elements are viewed independently, four decisions on inferences are necessary. The degree of risk for each inference varies across the elements. In judging populations, the researcher may have a sense that she can intuitively evaluate the riskiness of inference by getting to know a sample. Parameters and populations can be differentiated from constructs and environments, because in the former a researcher can develop some sense as to how at-risk she is, but not in the latter. That is, BASS researchers are probably more comfortable when experiment elements or theory elements are more like those of the physical sciences, such as neural action potentials, with any conclusion entailing less risk in the inference than with elements that are more BASS-like, such as intelligence.

Interestingly, theory elements expressed in more PS-like terms assure less riskiness in the basis for inference but greater riskiness in inferring directly from variables to constructs. An instance of the latter might be framed as, "Does the neural action potential correspond to behavior?" By distinction, theory elements that take on more behavioral science qualities have greater riskiness in developing the basis of inference but less for the actual inference. That is, only if one can establish that some variable captures intelligence can an inference about intelligence be made. However, once the basis has been assured, the inference is straightforward. It seems then that although there are many values in moving toward more PS-like indices, such a predilection seems to be accompanied by off-setting mounting costs.

An alternative interpretation of the differences among the elements employed to develop inference comes from changing the criterion from riskiness to satisfaction. A researcher can typically examine the observation units themselves for population membership criteria to make a judgment on her satisfaction with them. She cannot do so for parameters, but can take some comfort in setting tolerable risk levels given for an algorithm. The only way to satisfy herself about constructs is through indirect evidence given by validities and reliabilities. For environments, there are no historic means to arrive at satisfaction because the concern has not been examined.

Because environments are partially defined by constructs, it may be possible to use the assists available for other constructs, such as indices of reliability and validity, to increase topical or personal theory about their influence.

Yet an additional distinction segregating environment from the other theory elements, at least with human subjects, is that each observation unit can and may have an idiosyncratic perception. That is, each observation unit defines the salient features of the temporal, spatial, and social/affective context for self. Moreover, although the researcher may attempt to control the context through some framing mechanism(s), it is unclear that uniformity of perception by observation units can be achieved. More importantly, without expenditure of significant resources if even then, it will be unclear whether uniformity of perception has been achieved across sampling units.

It is probable that the modal response to this difficulty in determining perceptual consistency is some gross designation of the general spatial and perhaps temporal context(s). If the social or affective context is deemed important to the modeling of the experimenter, she may report her perception of it. In this approach, the variance of context appears as an inflator of the error term, diminishing the likelihood of obtaining significance for treatment(s). Alternatively, an experimenter could opt to sample environments by expending significantly greater resource to bring this theory element under more stringent experimental control. The latter choice appears to be made infrequently, which may reflect reasonable tacit knowledge of the importance of environment for the BASS or, alternatively, may explain some of the BASS difficulties in defining theories allowing generalization.

When and if environments become important to evolution of some personal theory, the element must be brought under experimental control. This is likely to be achieved by scaling the saliency of environment facets to make decisions about the perceptual inclusion or exclusion of each facet. If a researcher questions the relative or ordinal potency of environmental factors, comparisons yielding rank order for indexing potency may be worthwhile.

The above discussion is framed as though the elements are separable and independent. Although this approach eases examination of the untroubled ideal situation, more often the experiment is troubled because of the interaction of the elements or is potent because of their interaction. The vital areas for examination are both the consequences of obtaining the desired result and of obtaining an undesired result. Typically, behavioral scientists are interested in rejecting the null hypothesis because it is not consistent with the critical research hypothesis. We consider that very common case at length.

There is a transition from personal theory to experiment and, after the experiment, a transition returning to theory, and each transition occurs in two stages. The initial shift is from constructs to variables, with the operational definitions of the variables enabling formation of the testable null hypothesis. The experimental circumstances are then specified by reducing the other three theory elements to experimental realizations. In complementary fashion after the experiment, the inferences drawn for theory revision follow acceptance or rejection of the testable null hypothesis, first for populations and environments. When the experimenter has satisfied herself that the sampling, conditions and statistics of her inferences represent satisfactory realizations, she then draws the inferences on constructs leading to revision of her personal theory.

The Experiment Outcome Is Unexpected

The situation may be even less tidy when the probability value turns out to be greater than the Type I error tolerance. When this occurs, the researcher fails to reject the null hypothesis. The phrase "fail to reject the null hypothesis" does not provide evidence that the null hypothesis is true, which would presume that the treatment effect is completely absent in the population. When the probability is greater than α, it is crucial to identify an explanation or set of explanations for why the null hypothesis was not rejected, if a researcher hopes to advance her personal theory in a systematic fashion. Two fundamental questions govern the search for such an explanation; one is on the adequacy of the experiment and the other is on the adequacy of personal theory.

Experiment Adequacy

The explanation for a failure to reject the null hypothesis may result from one or more threats to the several validities of an experiment. For the most part, unexpected failure to reject the null hypothesis can be traced to problems with the precision of the experiment. Consider some examples:

1. It was determined that the presence of a video camera in the experiment room influenced subject behavior.
2. A second and unintended interpretation of the instructions to subjects is identified.

3. The room in which data were collected had a temperature problem that influenced some electronic circuitry used in the experiment.
4. The time resolution of a measuring device turns out to have been too gross.
5. Differential attrition rates occurred among the sample groups due to some aspect(s) of the treatment conditions.

In each case, the unanticipated threat to validity elevated the level of systematic experiment error or reduced the treatment effect and thus reduced the sensitivity of the experiment. As a result, the expected treatment effect or some variation of it was masked. If the researcher in any of these situations took an all-or-none view of the probability versus α outcome, the treatment effect would be overlooked entirely.

This is not to say that this same researcher should conclude that the treatment effect is present in the population. Clearly, no evidence to support such a statement is to be found in this context. However, an a posteriori, or after the fact, examination of the experiment validity would provide valuable clues about how to look for such evidence in some future experiment(s). That is, the experimenter would understand how to maximize hypothesis effects and minimize error effects in subsequent experiments.

A posteriori statistical power can assist the researcher in searching for an explanation for an unexpected failure to reject the null hypothesis. The a posteriori statistical power analysis differs from the a priori power analysis in that the observed sample estimates are employed in the necessary calculations. Recall that an a priori power analysis called for specification of the α level, the $1 - \beta$ level, and the magnitude of the effect size, so that the user could then solve for n. In the a posteriori power analysis, the researcher uses alpha, n and the observed effect size to solve for $1 - \beta$. Cohen (1988) provides power tables indexed by n, α, effect size and by degrees of freedom for a variety of statistics.

What is an explanation for unexpectedly low statistical power? An obvious answer is a smaller-than-expected effect size. Recall that during the course of an experiment, the researcher has absolute control over the alpha level, the $1 - \beta$ level and the sample size. The observed treatment effect, however, is outside her control, being determined wholly by the observational units. Given a satisfactory prior power analysis and a valid and precise experimental design, an unexpected failure to reject a null hypothesis is explained by the magnitude of the effect size.

When an effect size turns out to be smaller than expected, a researcher has two options. The first is to dismiss the observed treatment effect as trivial, given the prior criterion of experiment sensitivity. The smaller-than-expected response is much more likely to occur in confirmatory research, in which the accuracy of such definitions is specified with greater confidence.

The second option is to reconsider the criterion. On reflection, a researcher may decide that although the magnitude of an observed treatment effect was smaller than her estimate, the result is not trivial and does indeed constitute a worthwhile addition to the existing model. This decision implies that future experiments will require greater sensitivity in the form of larger sample sizes, all other matters presumed constant. Notice that the researcher is not in a position to conclude that the lesser treatment effect is a characteristic of the population. Such a conclusion must await the outcome of further investigation. The observed treatment effect is a sample-based observation that provides more than an improved estimate of the relationship between two or more parameters. As an outgrowth of the experiment, both the explanatory model and the researcher's understanding of the problem have expanded.

Theory-Based Adequacy

The prior section addressed the failure to reject the null hypothesis resulting from compromising the legitimacy of an experiment. This section addresses explanations of failures to reject the null hypothesis arising from constraints on the potency of one's personal theory. Examples include:

1. It is determined that the dimensionality of a construct had not been satisfactorily appreciated.
2. The population definition turns out to be too broad, with the resulting sample more heterogeneous than expected.
3. A relationship among dimensions of constructs becomes evident, giving rise to suppression of the treatment effect.
4. The negative implication of undifferentiated environments in a collection of theory statements becomes apparent.

In each case and in general, the result can be a diminution of the treatment effect or an inflation of the expected error or both. However, whether the result is expected or unexpected, only through continuing experimentation or, perhaps, through insightful modeling can the inadequacies of personal theory be revealed.

One of the motivations in writing this work is the authors' discomfort with the relationships between theory and experiment in the BASS. At this juncture we believe that the reader, having considered the examples and explanations of experiment-based failures to reject the null hypothesis plus the examples of theory-based failures to reject the null hypothesis, can readily understand the implications of the latter. But, both authors and reader having come so far, we cannot risk that these critical points in BASS theorizing be missed so, at the risk of redundancy, we continue with what we trust to be the obvious.

Programmatic research is a balancing act between precision in the explicitness of one's prediction and the likelihood that the prediction is wrong. Potency for theory revision is tied to explicitness of prediction among other things because, likely, the more specific the prediction, the more apparent a critical test. Therefore the experimenter should attempt to draw as explicit a prediction as she can. Narrow predictions come out of hard thinking. Given the complexities of BASS theory, however, more explicit predictions have higher probabilities of being unsustained.

Our belief is that unexpected results should occur often in the BASS. This view comes out of our perceptions that the complexities of the BASS, of the multidimensionality of constructs and environments, and of the complexities of the interactions of these elements do not foster sustainable explicit predictions. But in the face of these difficulties, we find merit in explicit prediction. Developing explicit predictions is even more difficult in the more exploratory phases of theory construction, yet we counsel their use anyway.

In the BASS, this implies that, first an experimenter should make as explicit predictions on experiment outcomes as she can. This should lead to the anticipation that some high proportion of experiment outcomes will be unexpected, that is, to fail to meet the predicted result. Most importantly, although it is necessary to examine experiment realizations to explain unexpected results, routine additional examination of the adequacy of one's personal theory is most likely to assist rapid theory advancement.

We believe programmatic research should be conducted through careful design and construction of experiments, the casting of specific predictions, and the re-examination of one's results, both expected and unexpected. In adopting the strategy of reaching for an explicit prediction and then being faced with an unexpected result, the researcher carefully examines her personal theory both before and after the experiment. By contrast, if she settles for the conservative route of choosing omnibus hypotheses when facing theoretical complexities, she need not confront theory carefully either before or after the experiment.

15

A Flow Chart for Experimentation

T he following chart summarizes the entire enterprise of experimentation, only some parts of which are covered in this book. The book's objective is to clarify the less transparent or more troubled facets of experimentation. The chart identifies the major points for decision in the process and the major tasks. The chart assist in identifying when tasks are to be done at a particular point in the process and affords a sense of proportion.

GIVEN some motivation for experimentation,
   IF, an experiment will enhance understanding, and:
      there is sufficient personal value in process or product or both to merit the
      undertaking;
      the costs of an experiment do not exceed the values,

   THEN:

LEVEL I ORGANIZING PERSONAL THEORY
   A. Conceptualizing personal theory

      What happenings (events) call for explanation?

> What is known from other accounts?
> What relationships can be discerned?

> What is known from my own observations?
> What relationships can be predicted?

> What observations do I believe are likely?
> What relationships do I purport?

      What do I believe accounts for the known observations?

   B. Developing personal theory
      1. Determine theory elements requiring clarification, assay literature and
          experience and distill essences of each theory element from both
          sources.
          a. Constructs: what internal attributes, traits, characteristics, etc.
              shape our understanding?
          b. Environments: what temporal, spatial, social/affective contexts
              influence the constructs?
          c. Parameters: what quantifications of theory elements or their inter-
              relationship are salient?
          d. Populations: what group of entities sharing (a) common (set of) fea-
              ture(s) embodies the constructs?
      2. Write theory statements
      3. Determine causal model(s)

LEVEL II. AUTHORING PERSONAL THEORIES

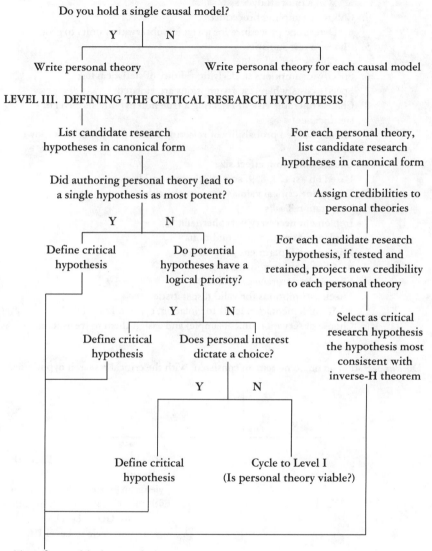

Do you hold a single causal model?

Y | N

Write personal theory   Write personal theory for each causal model

LEVEL III. DEFINING THE CRITICAL RESEARCH HYPOTHESIS

List candidate research hypotheses in canonical form

For each personal theory, list candidate research hypotheses in canonical form

Did authoring personal theory lead to a single hypothesis as most potent?

Assign credibilities to personal theories

Y | N

Define critical hypothesis

Do potential hypotheses have a logical priority?

For each candidate research hypothesis, if tested and retained, project new credibility to each personal theory

Y | N

Define critical hypothesis

Does personal interest dictate a choice?

Select as critical research hypothesis the hypothesis most consistent with inverse-H theorem

Y | N

Define critical hypothesis

Cycle to Level I (Is personal theory viable?)

Transform critical research hypothesis to H_p

LEVEL IV. DEFINING THE EXPERIMENT
  A. Planning Tasks
    1. Choose (valid & reliable) measures of independent and dependent variables
       a. Will a pilot study assist?
    2. Author the statistical hypotheses

   3. Choose the test condition(s)
      a. Will a pilot study assist?
   4. Choose a sampling procedure
      a. Determine procedure for assigning observation units to groups
   5. Choose a test statistic
      a. Choose critical value
   6. Specify assumptions underlying validity of statistical test
   7. Specify costs when test assumptions are violated
   8. Choose tolerable risk of rejecting a true null hypothesis (level of significance)
   9. Choose desired probability of rejecting a false null hypothesis (power of test)
  10. Choose minimum effect size
  11. Based on #s: 1, 5, 8, 9, and 10, choose sample size
  12. Determine critical value(s) for test algorithm
B. Implementation Tasks
   1. Implement necessary paraphernalia
   2. Implement experiment conditions
   3. Implement experiment procedures
      a. Choose subject instructions
   4. Choose data-storage procedures
   5. Check assumptions for valid test statistic
      a. If implementation leads to violation, cycle to Level IV, A5
   6. Choose observation units (sample) and assign them to treatments

Does expectation on outcome remain consistent with the critical research hypothesis?

Y | N

Re-examine Level IV. Then, IF alteration of any Level IV task yields an expectation consistent with the critical research hypothesis, GO to Level V; IF not, cycle to Level III.

LEVEL V. RUNNING THE EXPERIMENT
A. Execution Tasks
   1. Measure and record observations
   2. Check measures for accuracy and identify potential outliers

3. Compute descriptive statistics and estimate population parameters
4. Evaluate assumptions for test statistic

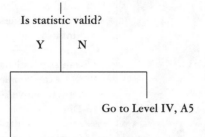

Is statistic valid?

Y | N

Go to Level IV, A5

5. Compute test statistic
6. Decide tenability of null hypotheses
7. Compute confidence interval(s)
8. Conduct a posteriori power analysis

LEVEL VI. EVALUATING THE RESULTS

Are results as expected?

Y | N

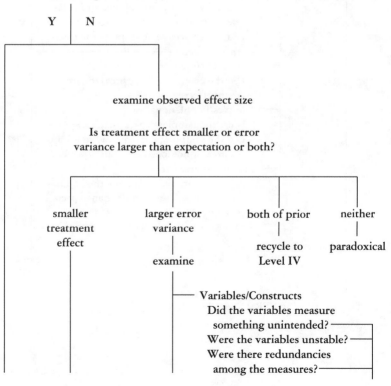

examine observed effect size

Is treatment effect smaller or error
variance larger than expectation or both?

smaller treatment effect   larger error variance   both of prior   neither

examine   recycle to Level IV   paradoxical

Variables/Constructs
Did the variables measure
something unintended?
Were the variables unstable?
Were there redundancies
among the measures?

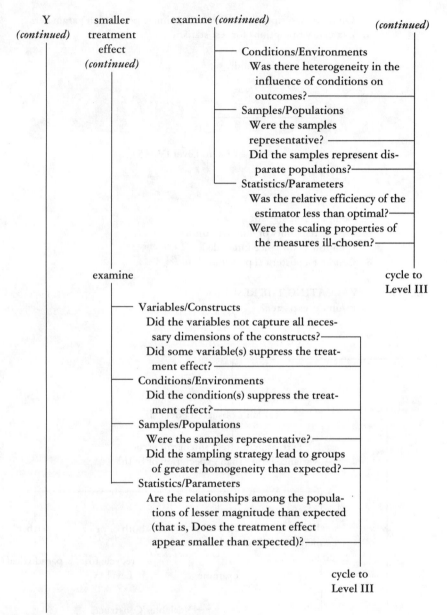

Y   smaller   examine *(continued)*   *(continued)*
(continued)   treatment
            effect   Conditions/Environments
            (continued)   Was there heterogeneity in the
                                                influence of conditions on
                                                outcomes?
                                            Samples/Populations
                                                Were the samples
                                                representative?
                                                Did the samples represent dis-
                                                parate populations?
                                            Statistics/Parameters
                                                Was the relative efficiency of the
                                                estimator less than optimal?
                                                Were the scaling properties of
                                                the measures ill-chosen?

            examine   cycle to
                                                                            Level III

                            Variables/Constructs
                                Did the variables not capture all neces-
                                sary dimensions of the constructs?
                                Did some variable(s) suppress the treat-
                                ment effect?
                            Conditions/Environments
                                Did the condition(s) suppress the treat-
                                ment effect?
                            Samples/Populations
                                Were the samples representative?
                                Did the sampling strategy lead to groups
                                of greater homogeneity than expected?
                            Statistics/Parameters
                                Are the relationships among the popula-
                                tions of lesser magnitude than expected
                                (that is, Does the treatment effect
                                appear smaller than expected)?

                                                                            cycle to
                                                                            Level III

LEVEL VII. REVISE PERSONAL THEORY

Section III

Introduction

The previous section detailed the particulars that optimize an experiment. We have argued that the potency of any experiment bears a direct relationship to the specificity of an experimenter's expectations of outcome. These expectations are best sharpened by raising one's sights from the needs of personal programmatic research to the broader concerns of the discipline. Moreover, greater impact on the discipline arises from such enhanced potency.

Section I organized the construction of a personal theory as an idiosyncratic combination of theory statements, interests, and speculations about causation. Section II focused on optimizing the development of new theory statements. As the body of theory statements enlarges, that is, as the evidentiary state increases, the explanations become more uniform, (i.e., less idiosyncratic) and tend to converge.

Section III examines how expectations are sharpened through research aimed at convergence. Chapter 16 establishes a probabilistic framework for applying the results of experiments toward construction of theory and toward unification or integration across theories. Chapter 17 examines the relationships among the results of experiments and causes-in-nature through the mediation of theory, with Section III providing a warrant for tying the conclusion of Section II to the beginning of Section I.

The book has provided the background necessary for the design and execution of influential studies. The background modeling of the

135

ideal has been developed and the compromises often encountered in realizing an experiment have been detailed. The explanatory hierarchy has been largely from personal theory to experiment result. The final chapters reverse the direction of the endeavor. By this point the researcher would have one or a series of results, each representing a theory statement developed from structured observation. The substance of Section III is accounting for the collected results—putting a causal model together, refining causal models, and selecting among competing causal models.

One disclaimer before examining the detail of bridging from experiment to personal theory: Everything in the previous section has been restricted to terms of the outcome of a single experiment. Ultimately, the destination is explanation of cause on the basis of the observed effect. That is, any experimenter is examining the null hypothesis and seeking inference about the prime hypothesis. That road is tortuous and, to stay with the metaphor, not taken in the light of previous experience, so that the route is not assuredly mapped from a single trip.

16

Systematic Theory Advancement

The long-range goal of all thought and study is a fuller understanding of ourselves and of the world that we inhabit. Formal theory expresses scientific understanding of the world, and theory is advanced incrementally on the basis of individual experiments. Section II concentrated on the deductive-like: general to specific portions of experimentation serving to enhance the value of ongoing experiments, progressively. We now consider the inductive-like: specific to general portions of experimentation. This chapter first describes the inductive-like processes that can optimize an experiment and then discusses how these same processes emerge from programmatic research to serve the evolution of causal models.

Inductive and Deductive Phases in Research

The experimenter conducting a research program cycles between experiment and theory. On the one side, she is designing and conducting experiments to put her insight and understanding to test and thereby to increase the sophistication of her personal theory. On the other side she is developing the ties within her personal theory that encapsulate her understanding so she can design ever more powerful experiments.

Chapter 5 concentrated on the arc of the research cycle from personal theory to critical research hypothesis. In that phase of the process, the experimenter particularizes from her single personal theory, or proposed causal model, to a specific expectation that becomes the critical research hypothesis. Most often, in that process, the experimenter desires a prediction that would be expected from her model but would not be predicted from alternative tenable causal models. That is, the procedures (1) are deductive-like in sequencing from general to specific and (2) involve a predilection for ruling out alternative candidate critical research hypotheses.

The focus is now on the arc of the research cycle that moves from the finding(s) of that experiment to the modeling of nature. Here, the finding, taken in the context of other theory statements, forms the basis for an inductive-like choice among competing personal theories. Unless faced with calamitous events, the experimenter adds one or more theory statements to each of her candidate personal theories, reconceptualizing each personal theory if she can, to encompass the growing set of theory statements.

Competing personal theories differ in the explanations of common or related sets of observations. Competing personal theories can be framed to be categorically distinct, as in the case of some characterizations of creationism versus evolution. However, the several personal theories are likely to share commonalities of explanation as well as of observation. As the sets of observations grow, so might the explanatory commonalities converge.

In contrast to the earlier-discussed portion of the deductive-like research cycling from theory to experiment, the procedures in this portion are more inductive-like in sequencing from specific results of individual experiments to more general causal models. Moreover, there is likely to be a predilection during these processes for ruling in rather than ruling out alternative models. That is, the experimenter entertains countercandidate personal theories as she seeks to unify her growing body of theory statements into a singular and most universal-like covering explanation.

The deductive-like processes of Chapter 5 for moving to a choice of critical research hypothesis are consonant with the logic and principles of testing hypotheses. The inductive-like processes for moving to the formation of more general causal models detailed here are not widely broadcast, neither are they routinely articulated nor addressed. We have, therefore, taken on the burden of providing a warrant specifically addressed to the relationship of the results of individual experiments and its impact on the development of causal models.

The Role of Induction in Organizing Theory

Watanabe (1960) develops the argument that results of research studies facilitate an inductive-like development of theory. Note that his use of "hypothesis" is equivalent to personal theory as defined herein. His discussion, therefore, applies to contrasting models of explanation, rather than contrasting research hypotheses within a personal theory.

Watanabe sets down ten criteria for inductive inference and its supporting evidentiary process. We believe that the formal process articulated by Watanabe has application uniformly across the BASS for developing topical theory as well as for unifying BASS theory. The ten conditions important to inductive inference are:

1. *A role for deductive inference*: "... inductive inference contains, as a necessary ingredient, a constant comparison of the deductive consequences from a hypothesis with the experiment" (p. 208). The first condition asserts that deductive inference plays a necessary role in inductive modeling. The deductive inference occurs during evaluation of the tenability of the research hypothesis, which is a statement of a general phenomenon on the basis of a single and specific experiment.

2. *Logical refutation by counter example*: "A hypothesis is disqualified when the hypothesis excludes the occurrence of a certain event ... while actual experience shows that this forbidden event in fact occurs .... This is the only part of the inductive process where deductive logic is the sole arbiter" (p. 209). If one's hypothesis asserts that X cannot occur and X occurs, the hypothesis must be rejected on this basis alone.

3. *A continuous measure of preferential confidence on hypotheses*: The essential theoretical difficulty in inductive inference is that with only finite evidence virtually no hypothesis is ruled out (except as in condition 2). For this reason, inductive inference is often held to be logically ill-founded. In applications of inductive inference, even though the inference cannot rule out any hypothesis, the researcher usually

prefers one or a few hypotheses because they best fit with the evidence. Indexing the fit requires a continuous measure of preferential confidence or CREDIBILITY (inductive probability) on each of the competing hypotheses (p. 209). Credibility is a measure of a subjective probability. It has no objective validity, but serves the purpose of indexing the plausibility of each of the hypotheses under consideration.

4. *A successive approach*: The essence of the scientific method resides "in successive improvement in knowledge . . . (T)heory [capitalization added] [must] be based on a procedure by which we 'modify' or 'improve' the evaluation of credibility in the measure as the body of evidence accumulates" (p. 209). A belief underpinning all scientific experimentation is that accumulating evidence makes explanation or theory a progressively better map of nature.

5. *The use of judgment from broader experience:* "A test of hypotheses [author note: Personal Theories] must be defined by some observational operation, and such a test must be instrumental in the above-mentioned successive improvement of the evaluation of the credibilities. However, in this actual evaluation, enough flexibility must be left to accommodate . . . a broader field of experience . . . to permit a unifying structure of a 'theory' covering a wide area of experience. Such broader consideration also serves greatly to invent new hypotheses as well as to degrade useless hypotheses before the test" (p. 209). Personal theories are evaluated by experiments and the experiment must make sense within one's general tutored knowledge of nature. Frequently, some new hypothesis may emerge or some considered hypothesis may be eliminated because of its congruity or incongruity with one's broader range of experience, and either occurrence can appropriately influence one's thinking at any time.

6. *A denial of absolute certainty for the validity of any hypothesis*: "No hypothesis [author note: Personal Theory] should be declared to be a law (i.e., credibility unity) on the basis of a finite number of observed data" (p. 209). Truth cannot be determined by induction.

7. *The existence of a law with objective validity*: Fundamental to any general scientific quest and independent of any preconceived judgment about any scientific hypothesis ". . . it must be guaranteed that some hypothesis, whether or not already considered, reaches credibility unity . . . [when] . . . the body of evidence becomes infinitely large" (p. 209). This condition is a statement of faith underlying scientific endeavor, asserting that nature is lawful and evidence will progressively accumulate that supports the true hypothesis.

8. *A distinction is maintained between credibility and confirmability*: ". . . credibility is the degree of preferential confidence . . . .

Distinct from credibility, there must be a certain measure of the degree to which a test, which is a series of the same type of observation, confirms a hypothesis individually taken, completely independent of the other hypotheses and of the experience outside the test in question" (p. 209). CONFIRMABILITY is conceptually distinct from credibility, though high confirmability must tend to increase the credibility. Watanabe differentiates credibility and confirmability to make the point that objective validity cannot be established through credibility but only through confirmability. Complete confirmability or a confirmability value of unity, as used by Watanabe, cannot be achieved as it is an ideal. The BASS approximate the ideal through application of the theory of probability. At the level of the individual experiment, confirmability is assessed through probability for statistical inference. With accumulated results, confirmability is assessed at the disciplinary level through application of the techniques of meta-analysis.

9. *The introduction of new hypotheses is allowed*: ". . . the model theory of induction must be such that we can add a new hypothesis at any stage of the process of induction and let it compete with other hypotheses which have already been considered" (p. 210). One's personal theory must always be open to a new hypothesis if it is supported by the data, that is, by the current theory statements.

10. *A state of anti-ergodicity and the applicability of the inverse H-theorem* (p. 210):

A. Ergodicity: An ERGODIC SYSTEM is one in which things, once disturbed, tend to return to their prior unorganized states, whereas things become progressively more organized in an anti-ergodic system when it is disturbed.

Watanabe's tenth condition holds that the mapping of the theory domain onto the nature domain will show anti-ergodicity.

B. Inverse H-theorem: The H-THEOREM expresses mathematically an increase of ENTROPY, or a breakdown in organization or structure, over time. In a typical ergodic, STOCHASTIC chain, the distribution of credibilities gradually spreads to all cases and the H-theorem shows an increase (or nondecrease) of entropy with time. In inductive inference, the distribution of credibilities becomes increasingly concentrated on a decreasing number of hypotheses—that is, it is anti-ergodic, so there must be an inverse H-theorem result, thereby showing a decrease or nonincrease of the entropy of one's induction with the growth of experience. The implications of the tenth condition are that theory building and theory unifying will be manifested as progressively larger credibilities that accrue to progressively smaller sets of personal theories. The H-theorem quantifies entropy and both credibility and confirmability provide measures of entropy.

What we take Watanabe to be saying is that, from the deductive-like side, one selects an observation and structures it to posture oneself for drawing some inductive-like conclusion(s) from the deductively-derived experiment. The researcher's goal is to be able to select among personal theories. Accordingly, a personal theory is not credible when an event *precluded* by the personal theory occurs as the outcome of an experiment. In all other cases, competing personal theories are assigned some degree of credibility that increases or diminishes with outcome. Credibility, then, can serve as an index of preference for or confidence in each personal theory as an explanatory model. The credibilities of the several personal theories sum to 1.0 and, in the ideal, a credibility of 1.0 assigned to a single personal theory labels it as "truth."

Because the credibilities are subjective weights, assigning initial values is difficult. A part of Watanabe's contribution is the recognition that the initial value does not matter but that quantification per se assists. Even more importantly, accumulating evidence drives the weights differentially in the direction of "truth." This last is a statement of faith.

In the absence of truth, the weights will be driven in favor of the personal theory that most closely approximates truth and this also is a statement of faith. Along the way, one knows that he is on the right track if (a) the personal theories continue to make sense within his broader experience and (b) if the process is progressively anti-ergodic.

Anti-ergodicism in causal modeling is facilitated by testing more specific rather than more general null hypotheses. That is, outcomes that are framed to be precise are likely to make large differences in a priori credibilities assigned to competing or even complementary personal theories, that is, to be anti-ergodic. Outcomes arising from the testing of omnibus null hypotheses are likely to result in reducing any differences in the a priori credibilities assigned to competing personal theories, that is, to increase the entropy and add to topical confusion.

Watanabe's use of credibility serves to provide an index on believability. Because we have not previously discussed credibility, but have stressed potency, the distinguishing characteristics of credibility and potency may not be clear. Potency refers to explanatory power rather than plausibility. That is, one might consider a series of scientific laws, recognizing that while each is credible, some are clearly more powerful than others.

The process offered by Watanabe transforms directly to Bayes' theorem for the situations where some explanatory scheme or schemes gain credibility from an experiment at the expense of others. Bayes' theorem, then, directly assists in assigning and manipulating credibilities among personal theories competing for place. By contrast, Bayes' theorem has *no* utility when one is considering alternative research hypotheses which are *not* formed to compete for place. The researcher retains the option of using the quantification available through Bayes' theorem so long as she is willing to frame her research hypotheses so that they are in direct competition.

The important insight from Watanabe's formulation is that there is a bootstrapping procedure for modeling causation on the basis of empirical evidence. The activity begins with some partially formed explanations or fuzzy general laws that are gradually refined by accumulating evidence. Further, it matters little in the long run how ill-formed the initial hypotheses or personal theories are, or how far off-base one's initial beliefs are. What Watanabe establishes is that the accumulating evidence will set the experimenter on the right path, even if her initial view is misguided. Watanabe's exposition fosters a quantitative process that in and of itself assists her in striving for universality of explanation.

17

Cause-Effect Relations

Chapter 1 framed the entire book, taking the reader to the starting point for viewing and understanding the architecture of experimentation. The route map acknowledged three domains—nature, theory, and experimentation—but the journey traversed the latter two only. We return to an examination of the relationships between the latter two and nature for two reasons. First, examining the relations among the three domains will highlight the original and central importance of the prime hypothesis (H_p). Second, the logic of experimental design becomes apparent as the alternate hypothesis and its predecessors, the critical research hypothesis and the prime hypothesis, are tracked across the domains.

The point was made early and repeatedly that some observation of nature motivates a study independently of whether the observation is within a stream of confirmatory research or is new—or newly framed—as in exploratory research. The observation piques a need for explanation or for confirmation of some explanatory scheme. Such an occurrence is not different in scientific endeavor than throughout other activities of daily living. The manner in which scientific enterprise does differ is in the formal process the researcher brings to constructing and bringing any exploratory scheme to test.

But first some reminders about—or, should you disagree, some arguments about—the three domains. Western science is grounded in a substantial belief in an objective reality. Scientific principles hold that nature has a physical existence independent of our perception. Further, there is the belief that some few recurring general principles form the key for rational analysis of objective reality. In addition, scientists believe there to be general principles that rationalize the sensing of that reality. While it is unclear how one would form the judgment, it may be argued that scientists have greater confidence in our general principles for nature than in our general principles for human sensation and perception.

However, there is no objective way to establish that there are general principles in nature—what we will call GOVERNING SYSTEMS—as, arguably, there is no objective way to establish that nature, itself, has an independent existence. But, if there is to be any scientific enterprise at all, one begins somewhere.

We begin with mind and with communication: Mind, because it is the creator and repository of intellectual process and structure; and communication, because it requires the apperception and encoding of organized forms of energy. From there we move without argument or warrant to acceptance of an objective nature and of a scientific enterprise. By the latter, we mean the belief in and pursuit of understanding of governing systems in nature. Science holds beliefs in general principles and in the advance of understanding through alternations of inductive-like and deductive-like inferences in combination with the acquisition of encoded forms of energy, that is, with communications from nature and from collegial scientists.

Given the above, what we infer about the governing systems in nature comprises a set of abstractions that themselves are an ideal or set of such ideals. These ideals constitute scientific laws. Whether or not there are governing systems in nature is unknown and unknowable but one either believes in such governing systems or stops trying to formulate scientific laws. Moreover, the human being can perceive only individual unique sensations and, rigorously considered, only sensations of difference or change. The search for any governing system in nature, then, must proceed through the induction of general principles abstracted from encoded and stored individual perceptions. Beyond perception of the individual sensations brought about by change or difference, one is necessarily in the domain of theory, though many philosophers of science hold that even perception itself is theory-laden (c.f., R. Hanson, 1958).

Untutored intellection about observations of nature organizes some primitive explanation. The scientific process, as it is practiced and as including the refinements herein proposed, is analogous but with significantly more detail. Like the untutored sequence, it also begins through the organization of some more or less primitive explanation. The explanations of science differ by being informed in two ways. First, they are canonical in form; that is, the explanatory scheme includes all four elements of theory and notes the dimensions and characteristics of each. Second, the state of knowledge about the general form and focus of any proposed explanation must be included, as must the data to be covered in the explanation. That is, the scientist's theorizing is influenced by the literature review that delivers inclusions and exclusions for the theory elements.

Additionally, a researcher gradually shapes an explanation as the basis for the eventual test. This evaluation process will require that each element of theory be realized in the experiment. The scientist's goals in the resulting experiment are to provide evidence for his candidate explanation and to rule out competing alternatives. The poorer the correspondence between theory and experiment elements, the less completely the experiment rules out alternative explanations. At the same time, on average, the better the correspondence, the more expensive the experiment will be.

The intellection combined with the prior knowledge taken from the literature review shapes the initial explanation progressively through more sophisticated research hypotheses to the critical research hypothesis. Recurringly, the researcher engages in dual considerations: What alternative explanations are ruled in and ruled out by the compromises necessary to realizing the ideal prime hypothesis? and What will be the likely resource costs of implementing each compromised prime hypothesis as a realized alternate hypothesis and finally as an experiment? All of the above occurs in the interface between nature as initial observation and personal theory as the evolving proposed explanation. The multiple stages and details of moving personal theory to empirical test provided the substance of the book.

Note that although we have separated out three domains, the outcome of the experiment as well as the experiment itself are parts of reality, parts of nature. Separating the experimental world as a domain apart from nature is useful because the experiment has a distilled quality about it. In moving from nature to theory and then from theory to experiment, the experimenter holds the four elemental categories to be necessary and sufficient, so that only these are realized empirically. When such an experiment yields an effect that corresponds to the initial observation or to the proposed consequent, particularly on repeated testing, the experimenter gains confidence in his understanding—in his now sophisticated explanation of the governing system in nature.

However, that explanation of the governing system in nature is no more than the evolved research hypothesis that gave rise sequentially to the prime hypothesis, to the realized alternate hypothesis, and to the null hypothesis formulated by negating the alternate.

The early parts of the process discussed above proceed from the reality-based observation within nature to the casting of the prime hypothesis in the domain of theory. Because the narrowing down and refinement of a primitive research hypothesis to the prime hypothesis is so much more content-based than the more process-based bridging from theory to experiment, this work has concentrated on the latter as process. That is to say, the essay has concentrated on theory to experiment rather than nature to theory, not because it is more critical but rather because there was more process to offer.

In sum then, the origins of theory are sometime observations of happenstantial events in nature. Although nature is composed of infinite complexities, the essence of nature is taken to be a small set of elements that are necessary and sufficient for capturing that reality. The elements are used to structure a microcosmic representation for systematic observations that allow the testing of theory. The worth of the structured observations for testing theory is in part a function of the quality of correspondence of the realized effect(s) to the earlier events in nature.

Developing the relationships between theory and experiment does not exclude nature as a domain requiring examination; rather it makes the examination systematic. We propose as a first approximation that the stages in cycling through the domains are something like the following:

A. Some observation(s) in nature gives rise to an initial explanation;
B. The explanation is formalized to one or more research hypotheses by providing canonical form for each;
C. The research hypotheses are informed from the literature review;
D. A critical research hypothesis is selected;
E. The critical research hypothesis is transformed to a prime hypothesis;
F. The alternate hypothesis is written as a best realizable approximation to the prime hypothesis;
G. The experiment is realized and the null hypothesis is tested:
   1. Is the effect what was purported?
   2. Did it occur for the reasons purported?

Once the initial observations of nature pique an initial explanation, the return to nature occurs in two forms: the recurring examination through the microcosm of the experiment and the opening at any time to new data that must be accommodated within the accepted explanatory scheme. Shy the latter, most scientific endeavor is the play between the formal structuring of theory and creating the microcosm of the experiment.

One can safely take the path proposed in the book as long as one maintains the necessity for scientific openness to new evidence from any source, the evidence bearing only its own witness. Further, the canons of experimentation require a Popperian (Popper, 1959) view that falsification of alternative explanations—of alternative proposals about the governing systems—and the ruling out of counter-explanations has as high a priority in experimental design and in programmatic research as initially establishing the explanation. Consideration of alternative explanations is the substance of the linkage between cause and effect, to which we now turn.

The present task is to illuminate the connections within the chain of reasoning linking cause and effect in scientific theory building. Cause is part of a relationship within theory that a researcher predicates. Cause links the elements of the theory statement through their internal ties to produce the theorized consequent of their interaction. That is to say, cause is a proposed map of the governing systems. It will operate through the elements of the personal theory to bring about some consequent (see Figure 17-1). The specification of the elements of the personal theory, in turn, specifies the characteristics of the consequent. A theory statement characterizes an outcome independent of cause. A consequent characterizes an outcome as a modeled interaction of all components.

Experimentation, by contrast, links the empirical realizations of the elements of a personal theory in an experimental interaction generating an effect. The effect is then rationalized by an *explanation*. The correspondences between the blueprint of nature that is the personal theory and the experiment, which is a model of reality built from the blueprint, are assured by the four validities. Evaluation of the validities warrants the correspondences and the utility of blueprint and model.

The Ties Linking Components of Theory

The chain of building theory, no matter the source of motivation or how initiated, becomes organized in the form of a disjunctive statement or syllogism—that is, the process is deductive. If the causal reasoning is deductively sound, then the interaction of elements of personal theory as specified yields a specified consequent (or change of state). As discussed in prior sections, parameters and populations must be defined and environments and constructs must be dimensionalized, with each dimension assigned a scale magnitude. All elements are ideally conceptualized in some initial set of circumstances and the consequent comes to pass of necessity, if the theory is sound.

The lawfulness of the BASS is captured in the theory statement as:

> Constructs, each of whatever dimensions and each being scalable in magnitude, distributed in one or more populations, under specified environmental circumstances, and quantified by a parameter, combining in a relationship yielding a consequent.

The content of the theory statement is governed by the causal relationship that is, itself, not expressed in the theory statement. The logical ordering for a visualization is, a cause preceding the particularized four elements and the predicted consequent, as seen in Figure 17-1.

The Empirical Chain of Experimentation

The reality-based empirical implementation has an analogous form, but its form is not required by deductive logic. There is no logical necessity because scientists cannot be assured about the governing system in nature and because of the variable influence of the operation of chance in sampling of observation units and of conditions. That is, this process is inductive-like. Each theoretical or ideal element is more or less well represented by its corresponding experiment element. The insightfulness, clarity, exactitude, and luck with which each theory

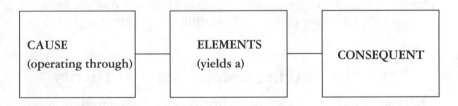

CAUSE	ELEMENTS	CONSEQUENT
(operating through)	(yields a)	

Figure 17–1 The chain of theory.

element is expressed as evaluated by the appropriate experiment validity determine the strength of the linkages between theory and experiment and, as a consequence, those between the cause in theory and the effect in experimentation. The empirical chain, realized in the transform of all theory components for the purpose of conducting an experiment, is expressed as:

> A set of variables, each having some range of values, distributed in the experimental sample under the specified conditions, and quantified by the statistics, yielding an effect, with the explanation imputed to be the governing relationship.

The progression, as illustrated in Figure 17-2, is from some initial state to a later state through an interaction among the experiment elements that is likely to be less than completely lawful in that it is subject to chance. The interaction results in an effect—some change in state—that is rationalized as lawful by means of an explanation.

The Relation of Effect and Cause

The two schema, of the theory and experiment chains of relationship, illustrate that cause is a unit of the chain of theory, and effect is a unit of the chain of experimentation. Tying effect to cause requires that the linkages in each chain be secure and that the theory elements be represented by corresponding isomorphic experiment elements, so that they are not under-, over-, or misrepresented. These

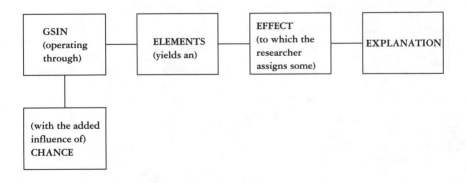

Figure 17–2   The chain of experimentation.

requirements are ideals, and because of the operation of chance are unachievable except by chance in any single experiment. The assertion of cause from effect in BASS theorizing is always inductive and, furthermore, as described by Watanabe (1960), the linkages are evidenced by progressively accumulating and converging data.

Juxtaposing the structural necessities of the two schema of Figures 17-1 and 17-2 illustrates the difficulties and the requirements for being able to warrant the modeling from effect to cause (Figure 17-3):

The top line of Figure 17-3 lays out the necessities of theory: Some presumed cause operates on the theorized essences of nature bringing about some theorized consequent. The second line shows the corresponding necessary units in the microcosm of the experiment as distilled by the experimenter. The experiment's impetus is derived from the dynamism and operational principles of nature, including the intrusion of chance. The dynamism brings about some change in the experiment elements or in their relationships, that is, some effect, and the experimenter offers an explanation. Of course, the explanation the researcher desires to promote is the causal statement from his personal theory.

What are the logical requirements that allow the researcher to assert his cause in personal theory as his explanation for the experiment? The requirements are, first, that the linkages within each chain are logically secure. Second, that there is isomorphism between the theory elements and the experiment elements. That is, the researcher

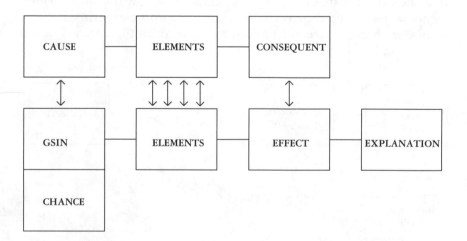

Figure 17–3   Building theory about nature through experimentation.

can conclude that the correspondences between each theorized element and its practical realization are of some arbitrarily high quality. Finally, third, that the effect in the experiment chain matches the predicted consequent in the theory chain—that is, the change in internal relations among the experiment elements in the experiment matches the change in internal relations among the theory elements predicted in the personal theory. Overall, the necessities are that the realization of the experiment has been conceptually and operationally good and that the operation of chance has neither misdirected the experiment nor diffused it. If the experimenter can have assurance that all three requirements are met, and given a match of effect with consequent, explanation can be synonymous with cause, thereby tying effect back to cause.

Earlier discussions have concentrated on the necessary sequence in realizing the experiment as moving from research hypothesis to alternate hypothesis and only then to the null hypothesis. Although the null hypothesis is necessary to the mathematical underpinnings for inferential algorithms, the logic of experimentation is grounded in the alternate hypothesis and not the null. The discussion immediately above has the same underlying logic and that logic holds much of the crux of experimentation. The theorizing behind empirical research and empirical research itself center on effects rather than the absence of effects. Although so much of the work of experimentation seems to involve the null hypothesis, null hypotheses are devices, albeit crucial, for determining the presence of effects within the tenets of scientific conservatism. Experiments are conceived to realize specific effects as confirming the researcher's observations and expectations about events in nature. Only through this route can theory be built to assist in understanding the patterning of nature.

References

Barcikowski, R. S. (1983). *Computer packages and research design* (Vols. 1-3). Lanham, MD: University Press of America.

Barnett, V., & Lewis, T. (1984). *Outliers in statistical data* (2nd ed.). New York: John Wiley and Sons.

Bayes, T. (1763). An essay toward solving a problem in the doctrine of chances. *Philosophical Transactions of the Royal Society, 53*, 370-418.

Buckingham, H., & Kertesz, A. (1976). *Neologistic jargon aphasia.* Amsterdam: Swets and Zeitlinger B. V.

Cohen, J. (1988). *Statistical power analysis for the behavioral sciences* (2nd ed.). Hillsdale, NJ: Lawrence Erlbaum.

Cook, T. D., & Campbell, D. T. (1979). *Quasi-experimentation: Design and analysis issues for field settings.* Boston: Houghton Mifflin.

Green, D. M., & Swets, J. A. (1966). *Signal detection theory and psychophysics.* New York: John Wiley and Sons.

Hanson, N. R. (1958). *Patterns of discovery.* Cambridge: Cambridge University Press.

Hopkins, K. D., & Glass, G. V. (1978). *Basic statistics for the behavioral sciences.* Englewood Cliffs, NJ: Prentice-Hall.

Kertesz, A., & Benson, D. (1970). Neologistic jargon: A clinicopathological study. *Cortex, 6*, 362-386.

Kroll, R. M., & Chase, L. J. (1975). A power-analytic assessment of recent research. *Journal of Communication Disorders, 8*, 237-247.

Marascuilo, L. A., & McSweeney, M. (1977). *Non-parametric and distribution-free methods for the social sciences.* Monterey, CA: Brooks/Cole.

Neyman, J. (1943). Basic ideas and some recent results of the theory of testing statistical hypotheses. *Journal of the Royal Statistical Society, 106*, 292-327.

Neyman, J., & Pearson, E. S. (1933). On the problem of the most efficient tests of statistical hypotheses. *Philosophical Transactions of the Royal Society of London, 231-A,* 289-337.

Oldfield, R. C. (1971). The assessment and analysis of handedness: The Edinburgh inventory. *Neuropsychologia, 9,* 97-113.

Popper, K. (1959). *The logic of scientific discovery.* New York: Basic Books.

Porch, B. (1974) *Porch Index of Communicative Ability in Children.* Palo Alto, CA: Consulting Psychologists Press.

Porch, B. (1981). *Porch index of communicative ability: Administration, scoring & interpretation* (Vol. 2, 3rd ed.). Palo Alto, CA: Consulting Psychologists Press.

Reese, T. W. (1943). The application of the theory of physical measurement to the measurement of psychological magnitudes, with three experimental examples. *Psychological Monographs, 55* (3), 1-88.

Schultz, M.C. (1973) The basics of speech pathology and audiology: Evaluation as the resolution of uncertainty. *Journal of Speech and Hearing Disorders, 38,* 147-155.

Stevens, S. S. (1951). Mathematics, measurement and psychophysics. In S. S. Stevens, *Handbook of experimental psychology* (pp.1-49). New York: Wiley.

Swets, J. A. (1964). *Signal detection and recognition by human observers: Contemporary readings.* New York: John Wiley and Sons.

Tanner, W.P., Jr., & Birdsall, T.G. (1964). Definitions of d' and η as psychological measures. *Journal of the Acoustical Society of America, 30,* 922-928. Reprinted in Swets (1964).

Tukey, J. W. (1977). *Experimental data analysis.* Reading, MA: Addison-Wesley.

Watanabe, S. (1960). Information-theoretical aspects of inductive and deductive inference. *IBM Journal of Research and Development, 4,* 208-231.

Glossary

α: A symbol signifying the probability of rejecting a true null hypothesis by chance alone, that is, the risk tolerance for committing a Type I error.

$1-\beta$: A symbol signifying the probability of rejecting a false null hypothesis, or unity minus the probability of failing to reject a false null hypothesis.

β: A symbol signifying the probability of failing to reject a false null hypothesis by chance alone, that is, the risk tolerance for committing a Type II error.

χ^2: A symbol signifying a family of inferential statistical tests of the equivalence of distributional densities.

δ: A symbol signifying a population effect size.

μ: A symbol signifying the mean of the distribution of an attribute of a population.

π: A symbol signifying a proportion of units in a population.

ρ: A symbol signifying a correlation coefficient between two dimensions or distributions of a population.

σ^2: A symbol signifying the variance of a population distribution.

H_0: A symbol signifying the null hypothesis.

H_A: A symbol signifying the alternate hypothesis.

H_P: A symbol signifying the prime hypothesis.

Accommodation strategy: The application of statistics that are minimally influenced by outliers and non-normal distributions, called robust statistics.

Algorithm: A statement in arithmetic notation; more generally, a mathematical formulation or equation.

Alternate Hypothesis: The transform of the prime hypothesis to the form representing the research hypothesis within the experiment or quasi-experiment; the transformation is achieved through operationalizing the constructs in the prime hypothesis as variables.

ANCOVA: An acronym for the analysis of covariance.

ANOVA: An acronym for the analysis of variance.

A posteriori: A Latin adjective or adverb (meaning: "after the fact") signifying one's knowledge about an experience gained through observation and inductive reasoning.

A priori: A Latin adjective or adverb (meaning: "before the fact") signifying one's knowledge about a prospective experience gained through deductive reasoning from known principles and accepted theory.

Arithmetic: Any of the operations of addition, subtraction, multiplication, and division. Arithmetic has been demonstrated (1) to express a set of logical relationships based in a system incorporating axioms and formal logic and (2) to correspond to nature.

Attribute: A property—quality, character, characteristic—naturally belonging to a person or thing.

Axiom: In formal logic or axiomatic systems, a proposition assumed without proof in order to study consequences from its application.

BASS: An acronym for the Behavioral and Social Sciences.

Bartlett's χ^2: An inferential statistic testing whether a population matrix has nonzero elements on the diagonal with zeroes elsewhere.

Box's M test: An inferential statistic for testing the multivariate analog of the assumption of homogeneity of variance for the univariate case.

Box-whisker plot: A procedure for graphical display of the sample data of a distribution in two-dimensional space.

Canonical: Rule-governed expression; a theory statement is canonical in making explicit mention of all four theory elements.

Canonical correlation: A multivariate inferential statistic for examining the independent–shared variances of two sets of data.

Categorization: The act of arranging entities in categories or classes on the basis of some defined set of characteristics used as the basis for determining that entities are identical or different.

Causation: The fifth component of theory, in addition to the four theory elements; the explanation of the dynamic relationships among the elements; an assertion of the governing system in nature serving to explain one's observations, including those made in experiments and quasi-experiments.

Cause: See Causation.

Component: One of the five constituents necessary to a theory or an experiment. Four of these correspond to essences of nature and are realizable; the fifth corresponds to the governing system.

Conditions: An experiment element; representing the theory element of environments.

Confirmability: The degree to which a test in and of itself (i.e., its probability for statistical inference) authenticates a personal theory. (See Credibility.)

Confirmatory research: Research within a more mature stage of knowledge or theory, often concentrating on confirmation of prediction.

Consequent: A term in the theory domain; the predicated outcome from the interaction of particularized theory elements linked to cause; an inference on the influence of cause in altering the relationships among the theory elements.

Consistency: In parameter estimation, the mathematical property of diminishing sampling error with increasing sample size.

Construct: An element of theory; property or process attributable to each observation unit of a population.

Construct validity: The fidelity of correspondence between a construct of the theory domain and one or more variables in an experiment or quasi-experiment; the integrity of representation of constructs as variables.

Contaminant: A data point taken from a distribution other than the salient one.

Correlation: An analysis technique yielding evidence about direction and degree of relationship between two dimensions of a population.

Credibility: A continuous subjective measure of preferential confidence or subjective probability in the authenticity of a personal theory. (See Confirmability.)

Critical research hypothesis: The research hypothesis formulated or chosen by the researcher to be put to test in an experiment as most critical to evaluation of personal theory.

Critical research question: An interrogatory statement expressing the dichotomous alternatives of a critical research hypothesis and its negation.

C: A robust alternative to analysis of variance as a test of statistical significance.

Deduction: A form of logic by which some generalization is applied to a specific instance; for example, because all men are mortal and Doe is a man, Doe is mortal.

Descriptive statistics: Mathematical indices intended to summarize or characterize data arising out of a sample of observation units.

Dimension: The quality of spatial extension. In scaling, units have dimensional properties of either a dichotomous—present or not present—or a continuously variable nature.

Disciplinary interest: The intellectual problems and concerns of the researchers in a discipline.

Discordancy test: A statistical procedure for identifying outliers in a set of data.

Discrimination: The act of distinguishing as different.

Disordinal interaction: An interaction among the values of the four cell means from two independent variables, each with two levels, constituting the presence of a reversal in rank ordering of the means for the left-hand column of one variable relative to the right-hand column.

Distribution-free statistic: An inferential statistic, analogous to a parametric statistic, but less stringent in its requirements for the distribution containing the parameter.

Domain: A field of action, thought, or influence.

Effect: A term in the experiment domain; the outcome of an experiment or quasi-experiment; the result of the governing system in nature operating on a particular combination of experiment elements.

Effect size: A standardized, that is, scale-free, index of the magnitude of a departure from a null hypothesis.

Efficiency: A mathematical property of estimators of parameters; the precision of an estimator relative to competing estimators in a comparison of the magnitudes of their standard errors.

Element (of theory or experiment): One of the set of realizable, necessary components, for example, the elements of an experiment or quasi-experiment are variables, conditions, statistics, and samples.

Entropy: The tendency of systems, in the absence of influence from externally derived energy, to show progressively less internal organization over time.

Environments: An element of theory; the temporal, physical, and social/affective contexts in which population members are observed during an experiment or quasi-experiment.

Ergodic system: A system in which things, once disturbed, tend to return to their prior, unorganized state.

Error term: In analysis of (co)variance, the denominator in the ratio of variance-attributable-to-the-independent-variable over residual variance.

Estimator: An algorithm derived to estimate the value of a parameter, given a sample of observations from the salient population.

Exact p value: In a prospective replication of an experiment, the probability of chance being responsible for a test result equal to or larger than that obtained in the experiment.

Experiment: A microcosm of the nature domain, capturing exemplars of the essences of nature, under circumstances allowing controlled observation. The choices of the exemplars are mediated by the theoretical model and typically allow control or intervention by the experimenter; a model of theory expressed as a microcosm of nature.

Experiment domain: A microcosm of the nature domain constructed or selected for the sole purpose of controlled observation as mediated by personal theory.

Experiment element: The elements of an experiment are variables, conditions, statistics, and samples. They are exemplars of the corresponding theory elements as captured in an experiment or quasi-experiment.

Exploratory data analysis (EDA): A collection of quantitative techniques used prior to application of inferential statistics for gaining a richer understanding of sampled data.

Exploratory research: Research within a more rudimentary state of knowledge or theory, often concentrating on explication of one or more elements of theory or on competing explanations.

Extensive dimension: A dimension underlying scaling on which attributes of observation units can be categorized, rank ordered and combined.

External validity: The fidelity of correspondence between both the population and environment elements in theory and the microcosmic representations of each as samples and conditions in an experiment or quasi-experiment.

Extreme score: The greatest or least in a distribution of sample values.

F_{max}: An inferential statistic testing whether a set of variances each estimate the same parameter.

Friedman *F* test: A nonparametric statistic for repeated measures data.

Full rank model: A statistical model in which the value of each sum of squares in regression analysis and in analyses of variance and covariance is adjusted for all other effects.

Governing system in nature (GSIN): The underlying regularities in nature which one attempts to capture as cause in theory.

H-theorem: A mathematical expression of the decrease in organization or increase in entropy in systems over time.

Induction: A form of logic by which one arrives at a general conclusion based on perceived similarities in specific instances; a means for arriving at some understanding of nature based on experiments and outcomes.

Inferential statistic: An algorithm yielding evidence about the likely quantitative characteristics of populations and their interrelationships.

Influential data point: Any data point that, when removed from the set, alters the interpretation of outcome.

Intensive dimension: A dimension underlying scaling on which the attributes of observation units can be categorized and rank ordered but cannot be combined.

Internal validity: The fidelity of correspondence between cause in theory and the explanation offered for the outcome of an experiment or quasi-experiment; the integrity of the face value of the experimental findings for revising theory relative to causation.

Interval scale (more properly: **equal-appearing-interval scale**): A scale for quantifying BASS phenomena in which the numerical intervals between categories are held to be equal.

Isomorphism: The state of two or more units that show a one-to-one relation in their elements or distinctive features.

Legitimacy: Refers to the quality of the correspondences of the elements of the experiment to the elements of theory.

Likelihood ratio: Ratio of the ordinates of two overlapping distributions at some defined value of the decision variable, that is, of the variable being displayed on the abscissa.

MANCOVA: An acronym for the multivariate analysis of covariance.

MANOVA: An acronym for the multivariate analysis of variance.

Mauchly's likelihood ratio criterion: An inferential statistic for testing if a matrix is equal to the product of an identity matrix multiplied by a constant.

Mean: The arithmetic average of a set of numbers; an index of central tendency.

Median: An index of central tendency, that is, the 50th percentile, founded in the rank ordering of data rather than in their arithmetic properties.

Mensuration: The act, process, art or an instance of measuring.

Multivariate regression: A single regression equation comprising multiple predicted variables.

Nature: The external world, presumed to exist independently of one's perception but including one's presence and influence. Nature can be described as comprising important characteristics (essences) and incidental characteristics, only the former being necessary for scientific understanding.

Nature domain: All that is apparently real, including self.

Nominal scale: Arguably the most rudimentary scale for categorizing observations; its requirements are that (1) like things, those sharing the defining characteristics, be categorized together; (2) like things be differentiated from unlike things, that is, those not sharing the defining characteristics; and (3) that categories have different assigned labels.

Nonparametric statistic: A inferential statistic testing a parameter in a distribution related to but different from the salient distribution.

Normal science: Scientific endeavor motivated to enhance the development of theory but not to modify it radically or lead to rejection of it.

Null hypothesis: The negation of the alternate hypothesis; the hypothesis tested in the experiment or quasi-experiment.

Number: A numeric symbol assigned to some attribute that meets all arithmetic requirements in magnitude.

Numeral: A numeric symbol assigned to some attribute in the absence of the requirement for meeting all properties of numbers.

One-tailed test: A procedure employing an inferential statistic testing a null hypothesis negating a unidirectional alternate hypothesis.

Operational definition: details the specific procedures followed in realizing a theory element as its corresponding experiment element, thereby determining the fidelity of correspondence and making a public report of the procedures.

Ordinal interaction: In a two-dimensional plot of two independent variables, each with two levels, a common rank ordering of the levels of the two variables.

Ordinal or rank order scale: A scale for quantifying BASS phenomena in which observations are clustered in categories which are ordered by magnitude of the defining characteristic.

Outlier: A data point that is remarkable in its isolation from the characteristic grouping of data points in the set.

Parameter: An element of theory; the medium for quantification, indexing magnitudes of constructs, as influenced by environments, or of relations among them.

Parametric test: An inferential statistic written to yield evidence for a decision involving a parameter of the population distribution and therefore involving assumptions about the mathematical properties of the distribution.

Perception: The hypothesis accepted by the individual on the basis of some decision(s) about an input.

Personal theory: A collection of theory statements relating to the researcher's interests, each weighted by its importance for the researcher's proposed explanation, plus the explanation of relationships or proposed cause in which the researcher chooses to invest. A personal theory must account for all valid and germane observations, contain a causal model and provide the basis for meaningful and testable hypotheses.

Pilot study: A preliminary endeavor to identify or select an experiment element or elements.

Point-biserial coefficient: An inferential statistic for testing the relationship between two variables when one is continuous and the other is dichotomous.

Population: An element of theory; the totality of entities or observation units sharing a common feature or set of features (constructs and environments).

Positivism: A philosophical system of Comte basing all knowledge on the positive (assured) methods of the physical sciences. Subsequently, an outgrowth called logical positivism posited a central doctrine that any proposition, except for analytic propositions, is meaningful if, but only if, it can be verified through an empirical procedure for deciding if it is true or false.

Positivistic science: Scientific endeavor within a positivistic philosophical position, asserting that there is an objective reality operating through general principles that are ascertainable.

Post hoc: A Latin term meaning after or subsequent.

Potency: Refers to the quality of the correspondences of the elements of theory to the essences of nature, or to the utility of these correspondences for explanation.

Prime hypothesis: A canonical statement; the mathematical equivalent of the critical research hypothesis expressing a proposed consequent from personal theory.

PS: An acronym for the Physical Sciences, considered as a whole and differentiated from the behavioral and social sciences.

Quasi-experiment: A microcosm of nature where one or more experiment elements are beyond the experimenter's control, but with controlled observation possible.

Rank order scale: See Ordinal scale.

Ratio scale: A scale for quantifying BASS phenomena having arithmetic properties.

Relative efficiency: Relative magnitudes of sampling errors among competing estimators.

Research hypothesis: A prospective theory statement; canonical in form.

Research question: An interrogatory statement offering the dichotomous choice of the assertion and negation of a research hypothesis.

Research statements: The pair of statements comprising a research hypothesis and its complementary research question.

Response behaviors: The actions, activities or behaviors that can be quantified in experiments and quasi-experiments for purposes of testing hypotheses.

Robust statistic: An inferential statistic unaffected by outliers.

Sample: An experiment element; a representation of a population as a set of observation units in an experiment or quasi-experiment.

Sampling: The act of selecting observation units from a population for participation in an experiment.

Scaling: The assignment of numerals to the attributes of a population or sample according to a set of rules.

Sequential entry model: A statistical model used in regression analyses and ANOVAs wherein the ordering of effects is prescribed and the sums of squares for each entry are adjusted for all preceding effects.

Signal: Some change in nature that can be defined or characterized by its physical attributes.

Sign test: An inferential statistic for the tenability of equality of proportions for a dichotomous outcome variable in an experiment.

Standard error: The standard deviation of a sampling distribution.

Statistic: An experiment element; a representation of a parameter in an experiment or quasi-experiment.

Statistical conclusion validity: The fidelity of correspondence between the parameter element in theory and its representation as one or more statistics in an experiment; the integrity of parameter estimation.

Statistical hypotheses: The two hypotheses realized and tested in an experiment; the null and alternate hypotheses.

Statistical power: The probability of rejecting a false null hypothesis. From an a priori perspective, $1-\beta$ is the power desired for a particular analysis; an a posteriori save analysis of $1-\beta$ yields the statistical power that one could expect in a faithful reproduction of an experiment.

Stem and leaf display: A two-dimensional tabular presentation of all scores in a sample of data.

Stimulus: Those portions of a signal to which an observation unit is sensitive.

Stochastic: A process involving a sequence determined randomly rather than by rule.

Theory: A system for modeling nature conceptually through its essences, combining observations to be rationalized within a generalized explanation including a causal model. A map of nature. The components of theory are four elements, each expressing an essence of nature, and a fifth component, cause, capturing the relationship among the elements.

Theory component: Theory organizes explanations of nature as comprising five components, which are the four theory elements plus cause.

Theory domain: All that is in the ideal, including but not limited to personal theory.

Theory element: A theory element captures an essence of nature but not its governing system. The four theory elements are constructs, environments, parameters, and populations.

Theory statement: Canonical statement (explicitly mentioning all four theory elements) of the relations among theory elements relative to an observation (within an experiment or quasi-experiment) without mention of cause. A theory statement is formed in an active, declarative voice and its negation must be empirically testable.

Topical theory: A generally accepted personal theory, representing the accepted set of theory statements plus the predominant explanation, within a discipline.

True experiment: See Experiment.

Two-tailed test: A procedure employing an inferential statistic for the tenability of a null hypothesis negating a two-sided alternate hypothesis.

Type I error: The probability of rejecting a true null hypothesis on the basis of chance alone.

Type II error: The probability of failing to reject a false null hypothesis on the basis of chance alone.

Unbiasedness: The mathematical property of fidelity in parameter estimation; neither systematic overestimation nor underestimation.

Unweighted mean: The arithmetic mean of one or more levels of some dimension which is uninfluenced by the sample size at each level.

Validity: Consonance of components of the experiment and theory domains.

Variable: An experiment element; a representation of a construct in an experiment.

Weighted mean: The arithmetic mean of two or more levels of some dimension calculated to include the influence of the sample sizes at each level.

Wilcoxan's matched-pairs test: An inferential statistic that is a more powerful alternative to the Sign test.

Windsorized mean: An arithmetic mean calculated after the extreme scores are replaced with the values of their nearest neighbors.

Index

167